NCLEX Strategy & Pharmacology Review Book:

Nursing Review Book For Answering Prioritization & Next Generation Questions

By

Julie Chinwe Anyanwu RN, NPCH, MSN

DORRANCE
PUBLISHING CO
EST. 1920
PITTSBURGH, PENNSYLVANIA 15238

Dorrance Publishing Co
585 Alpha Drive
Suite 103
Pittsburgh, PA 15238
Visit our website at *www.dorrancebookstore.com*

ISBN: 979-8-89211-149-2
eISBN: 979-8-89211-647-3

This NCLEX strategy and pharmacology book is dedicated to God Almighty. God inspired me, and I am thankful for God's guidance, strength, and mercy throughout my studies. This is God's vision to me from Habakkuk 2:2: "Write the vision and make it plain on tablets, that he may run who reads it." I believe that this book is a gift from God and will be a blessing to many students. I pray that it will be used to help all nursing students pass the NCLEX.

I am humbled and grateful for the opportunity to share my knowledge with others. I ask for His guidance and protection for all those who will read this book. May they succeed in their studies and achieve their goals. Amen.

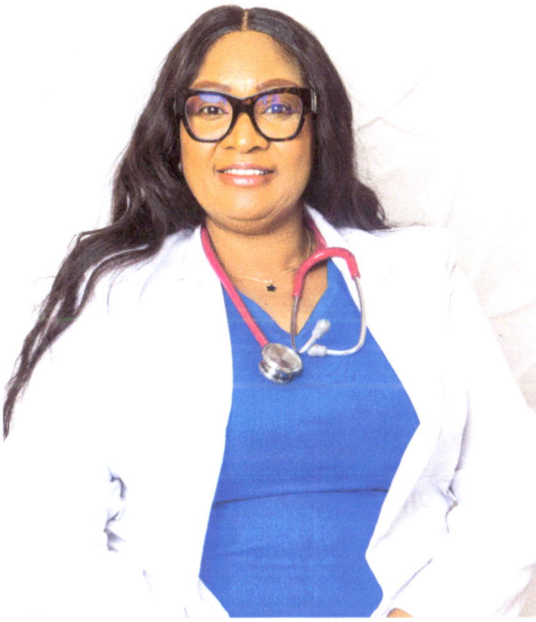

It is every nursing student's dream to obtain their license as soon as possible after completing nursing school. Unfortunately, some students struggle with the NCLEX exam before passing. The NCLEX exam is a rigorous test that requires students to demonstrate their knowledge and skills in nursing. It can be a difficult test for students who have spent time and effort learning the material. Nursing students seek help from professionals such as NCLEX tutors and counselors to prepare and pass.

I am passionate about making a positive impact on students, and this is why I created this JACKS NCLEX REVIEW. As a former nursing student who has the zeal and patience to learn nursing content and strategies to pass the NCLEX, I can assist nursing students who are struggling to pass the NCLEX. I strive to provide a comprehensive NCLEX review course that helps students understand the NCLEX format, Case Study, the content, and the strategies to prepare them for the NCLEX. I am committed to providing the highest quality NCLEX review materials and resources tailored to nursing students' needs. I am confident that this Jacks NCLEX Review book will enable nursing students pass the NCLEX. I am dedicated to helping students reach their nursing goals. My NCLEX review course is designed to assist nursing students succeed and reach their goals. I am confident that this course will be an invaluable asset to students preparing for the NCLEX.

We are pleased to welcome you to Jacks NCLEX Review, where students can learn the strategies they need to pass the NCLEX. My name is Julie Chinwe Anyanwu RN, MSN, NCPH. I am author and instructor of this *NCLEX Strategy and Pharmacology Review Book*. This review offers students a comprehensive overview of the NCLEX examination. It covers topics such as how to answer nursing content questions, NCLEX question types, NCLEX strategies, NCLEX practice questions, and pharmacology review. It also provides helpful resources and support to help students succeed.

I wrote this NCLEX Strategy review book under the inspiration of God Almighty. God called me an "NCLEX instructor." I was surprised and delighted to learn of this new opportunity. I knew that I had the ability to teach others and I was excited to be able to use my knowledge and experience to help future nurses. I was confident that this was going to be a great journey by God's grace. It happened while I was studying. God gave me the courage to take the NCLEX and pass so I could impact others with that knowledge. As God spoke to me at least three times, He urged me to study quickly and succeed. Additionally, he told me that many students need my assistance to be their instructors. Today, I coach nursing students to pass their NCLEX exams as an NCLEX instructor.

JACKS NCLEX REVIEW

I am truly grateful for God's guidance and support. Being able to assist nursing students in achieving their goals is a blessing for me. There is nothing more rewarding to me than seeing nursing students and repeat test takers who have joined my review program pass the NCLEX on their first attempt and become successful nurses. This NCLEX Strategy review book is intended to help those preparing for the NCLEX exam. I pray that it will be a source of inspiration and guidance to those in need. I also hope that it will be a source of comfort and reassurance to those who are feeling anxious or overwhelmed. May God be with you all and may you succeed on your journey.

I know that some students find the NCLEX exam challenging. This NCLEX Strategy review book will help you prepare for your examination. It will help you understand the review of nursing contents, case study questions, practice answering prioritization questions, and gain the confidence to pass the exam. The book also covers topics such as time management, test-taking strategies, and stress management. It is an essential resource for any student preparing for the NCLEX. "Because passing your NCLEX is your number one goal." This *NCLEX Strategy and Pharmacology review book* will surely simplify your study and YOU WILL PASS NCLEX BY GOD'S GRACE!

SCAN ME

TABLE OF CONTENTS

PART 1

PART 2

PART 3

ASSESSMENT VS IMPLEMENTATION STRATEGY

Assessment is the process of establishing a data profile about the client and his or her health problems. The nurse obtains subjective and objective data in several ways: talking to clients, observing clients and/or significant others, taking a health history, performing a physical examination, evaluating lab results, and collaborating with other members of the health care team. Once you collect the data, you compare it to the client's baseline or normal values.

However, on the NCLEX-RN® exam, you will be given a clinical situation and asked to establish priorities. The possible answer choices will include both the correct assessment and implementation for this clinical situation. The strategy to choose the correct answer when both the correct assessment and implementation are given. Think about these two steps of the nursing process assessment and implementation.

Assessment is the process of establishing a data profile about the client and his or her health problems. The nurse obtains subjective and objective data in several ways: talking to clients, observing clients and/or significant others, taking a health history, performing a physical examination, evaluating lab results, and collaborating with other members of the health care team. Once you collect the data, you compare it to the client's baseline or normal values. On the NCLEX-RN® exam, the client's baseline may not be given, but the knowledge you gained in nursing school will help you attempt the question. On this exam, you are expected to compare the client information you are given to the "normal" values learned from your nursing textbooks.

Assessment is the first step of the nursing process and takes priority over all other steps. It is essential that you complete the assessment phase of the nursing process before you implement nursing activities.

Types of Assessment: Subjective and objective assessment data

a. **Subjective:** an assessment that cannot be measured or measurable. Think of what the client says! For example, the client says, "I am cold or warm." The nurse asked the client to rate the pain using the FACES Scale. The FACES scale is a visual tool for assessing pain in children and others who cannot quantify the severity of their pain on a scale of zero to ten.

b. **Objective**: an assessment that the nurse collected that has measurable data. Also, objective data is data that is collected or obtained via established or verifiable facts and sources. It is collected to confirm your suspicions and assumptions—or merely to gather dependable information.

Example: The nurse uses the sphygmomanometer to check the BP level of the client.

Implementation: Implementation is the care you provide to your clients. Implementation does not give information.

Actualization or carrying out the plan of care through nursing interventions.

Let us look at some questions that deal with assessment vs implementation in the nursing process.

When the question is a prioritization question, you will see the question like **"First, Essential, Most Importantly, Initially, Best, Highest Priority, Immediately, Primary, Next, Vital"** and then use the elimination process to answer or pick the correct answer from the options.

NURSING PROCESS

- **Assessment** **A**
- **Diagnosis** **D**
- **Planning** **P**
- **Implementation** **I**
- **Evaluation** **E**

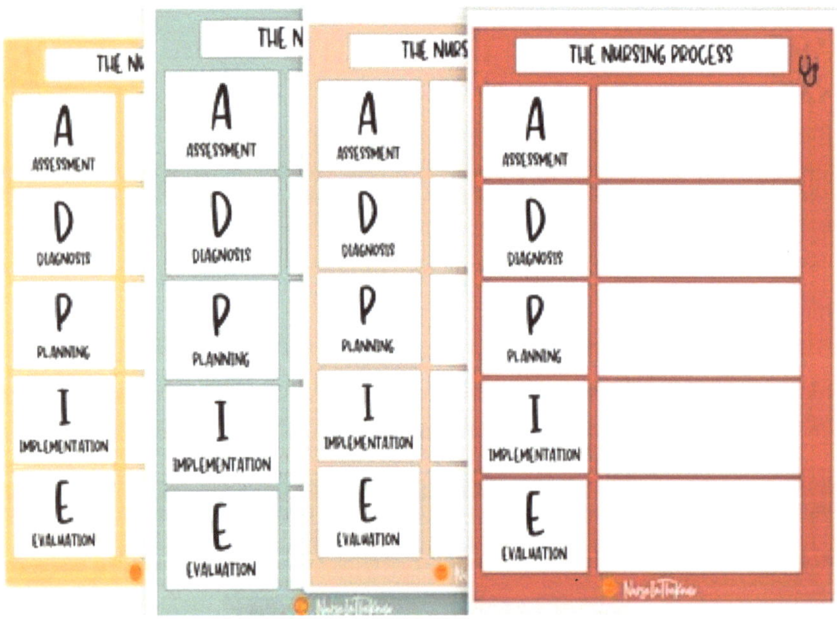

ADPIE is an acronym for the assessment, diagnosis, planning, implementation, and evaluation phases of a nursing intervention. It is a framework used by nurses to plan and assess patient care. The ADPIE model helps nurses to develop a plan of care that is tailored to the individual patient's needs. The ADPIE model also helps nurses to track progress and evaluate the effectiveness of the nursing care plan. The model is used as a guide to ensure that the patient's needs are being met and that the patient's health is improving.

NURSING DIAGNOSIS

The process of assessing potential or actual health problems, including those pertaining to an individual patient, a family, or community that fall within the scope of nursing practice; a judgment or conclusion reached because of such assessment or derived from assessment data. See also: **Diagnosis example:**

1. A nurse provides care to a three-year-old client who presents to the ER with a high fever, sore red throat, and drooling. Which of the following nursing interventions is the **priority**?

    1. Assess oral temperature immediately.
    2. Assess for the presence of stridor.
    3. Assess oxygen saturation.
    4. Position the client in the supine position.

To analyze the above question, follow the listed strategies:

- Pick the keywords from the question.
- Analyze the question in your own words using the critical thinking method.
- Then go to the option and use the elimination method to eliminate the wrong options.
- Use assessment vs implementation whenever there is a mixture of assessment and implementation.
- Compare the last two remaining options with the question before you make your final decision and pick your answer.

    1. Assess oral temperature immediately. Assessment
    2. Assess the presence of stridor. Assessment
    3. Assess oxygen saturation. Assessment
    4. Position the client in the supine position. Implementation

Rationale: Using the elimination process, option four is wrong because positioning cannot help this client who has epiglottitis. Then options one, two, and three all have an assessment to them. Now, go back to the question and find the option that has nursing intervention that is the priority. The correct answer is option two.

2. A client has been diagnosed with a UTI and is experiencing acute pain and comfort. **What should the nurse implement first?**

    1. Give pain medication as per the doctor's order.
    2. Encourage the client to increase oral intake of fluids.
    3. Notify the health care provider (HCP).
    4. Assess the level of pain using a pain scale.

To analyze the above question, follow the listed strategies:

Pick the keywords from the question.

Analyze the question in your own words using the critical thinking method.
Then go to the option and use the elimination method to eliminate the wrong options.
Use assessment vs implementation whenever there is a mixture of assessment and implementation.
Compare the last two remaining options with the question before you make your final decision and pick your answer.

3. Which action should the nurse implement for the client with a hemothorax who has a right-sided chest tube with vigorous bubbling in the suction control chamber?

1. Check the amount of wall suction being applied. Correct
2. Assess the tubing for any blood clots.
3. Strip the tubing proximal to distal.
4. Encourage the client to cough forcefully.

To analyze the above question, follow the listed strategies:

- Pick the keywords from the question.
- Analyze the question in your own words using the critical thinking method.
- Then go to the option and use the elimination method to eliminate the wrong options.
- Use assessment vs implementation whenever there is a mixture of assessment and implementation.
- Compare the last two remaining options with the question before you make your final decision and pick your answer.

Check the amount of wall suction being applied. Assessment
Assess the tubing for any blood clots. Assessment
Strip the tubing proximal to distal. Implementation
Encourage the client to cough forcefully. Implementation

Analysis/explanation of the question

Just because the question mentioned "implementation" does not mean that the answer will be an implementation in the nursing process.
Use your nursing school knowledge and ask yourself a question if you see bubbling in the suction control chamber is it okay? In this instance, it depends on the situation. Because it says, "vigorous bubbling." But in the suction control chamber, we should always see "gentle bubbling."
Use critical thinking to analyze the answer.
Answer options: Use the assessment vs implementation strategy to choose the right answer.
Check the amount of wall suction being applied. This is an assessment.
Assess the tubing for any blood clots. This is an assessment.
Strip the tubing proximal to distal. This is an implementation.
Encourage the client to cough forcefully. This is an implementation.

Rationale: Use an elimination process to eliminate the wrong answer option. From the scenario, options two, three, and four are eliminated because the options do not relate to what the nurse should do to help the patient. The correct answer is option one.

EXCEPTION TO THE RULE OF ASSESSMENT VS IMPLEMENTATION

There are some situations whereby the client will be in an emergency condition. In this situation, the nurse must assess first before implementing. A situation where:

- The client, either an adult, infant, or child is in distress/emergency.
- Ask the client, "Are you okay?"
- Check pulse if no pulse! Then start **CPR** immediately!
- Ask someone to call 911.
- Thirty chest compressions
- Two rescue breaths
- Repeat until an ambulance or automated external defibrillator (AED) arrives.

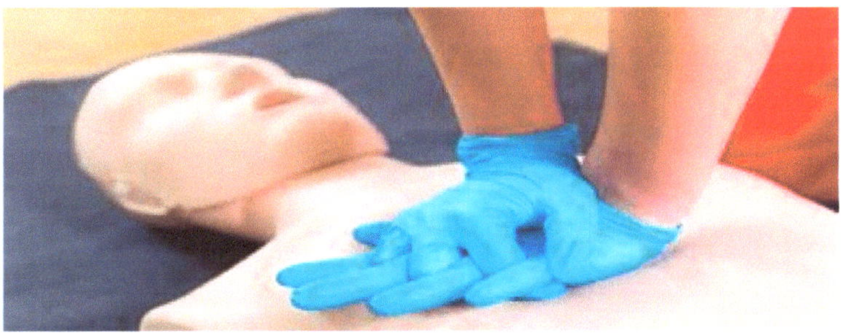

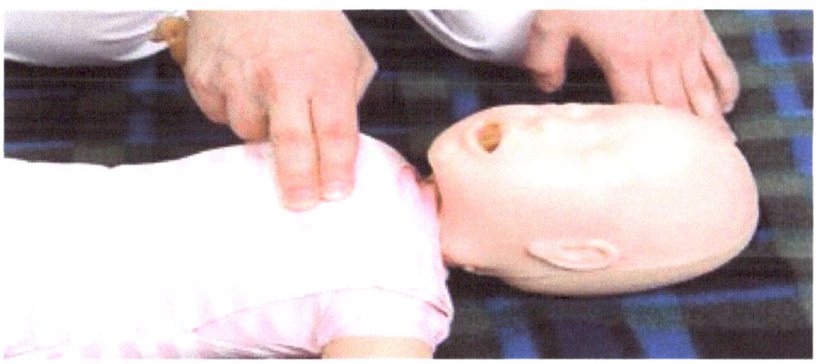

CHOKING CLIENT

Choking happens when an object lodges in the throat or a windpipe blocking the flow of air. Watch for these signs of choking:

- One or both hands clutched to the throat
- A look of panic, shock, or confusion
- Inability to talk

- Strained or noisy breathing
- Squeaky sounds when trying to breathe
- Cough, which may either be weak or forceful
- Skin, lips, and nails that change color, turning blue or gray
- Loss of consciousness
- If a choking person can cough forcefully, let the person keep coughing.
- Coughing might naturally remove the stuck object.
- If a person can't cough, talk, cry, or laugh forcefully, give first aid to the person.

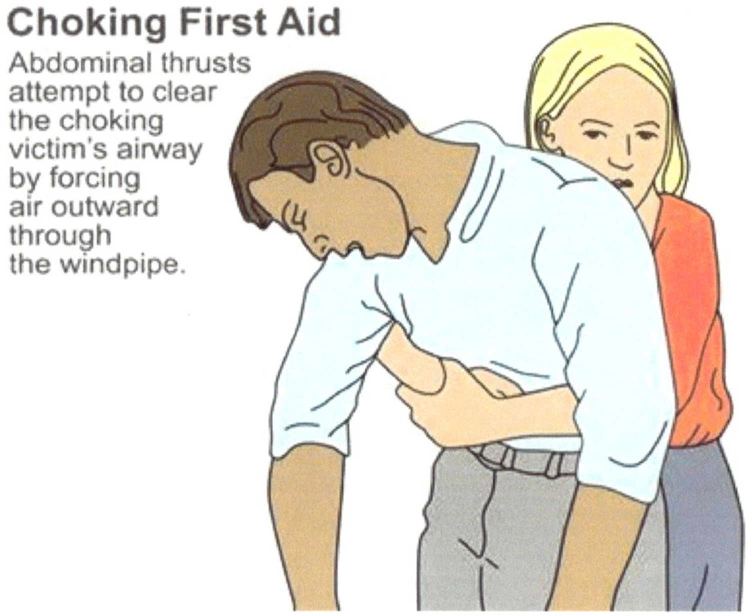

Heimlich Maneuver: What should I do before I start the Heimlich maneuver?

- Ask the person if he is choking.
- If he nods yes, ask if he can speak.
- **Call 911 if the person cannot speak.**
- You can then perform the Heimlich maneuver on the person until help arrives.
- If he can speak, this means his airway is only partly blocked.
- Tell the person to try and cough to push the object out of his airway.

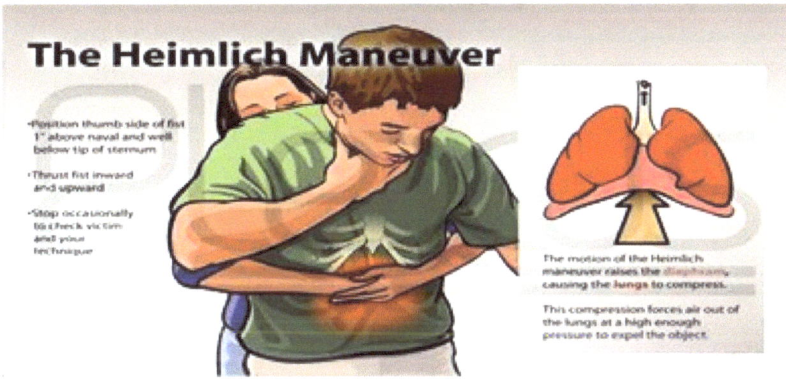

NCLEX Style Question?

When should you not use the Heimlich maneuver?

If the person is unconscious. In this scenario, start CPR immediately and have someone call 911 to get immediate medical attention.

INSERTION AND REMOVAL OF TRACHEOSTOMY TUBE

Insertion of tracheostomy tube: It is important you know the method of inserting and removing the tracheostomy tube. The surgery to insert a tube in the trachea is called a tracheostomy. The surgeon makes an opening, called a stoma, in the front of the neck, below the larynx. The surgeon puts a curved plastic tube called a tracheostomy tube into the stoma.

Why should a patient be place on trach:

Reason could be unsteady airway (floppy airway), due to lack of developed tracheomalacia.

Ineffective airway due to blockage know as tracheal stenosis.

As a result of Trauma-surgery, or tracheal separation.

When should you suction patient on a trach? Trach should be suctioned only when the patient needs suctioning. Avoid over-suctioning as it causes more problem and secretion to the patient.

Trach should be cleaned with soap and water, or hydrogen peroxide, or other cleanser on daily bases and as needed.

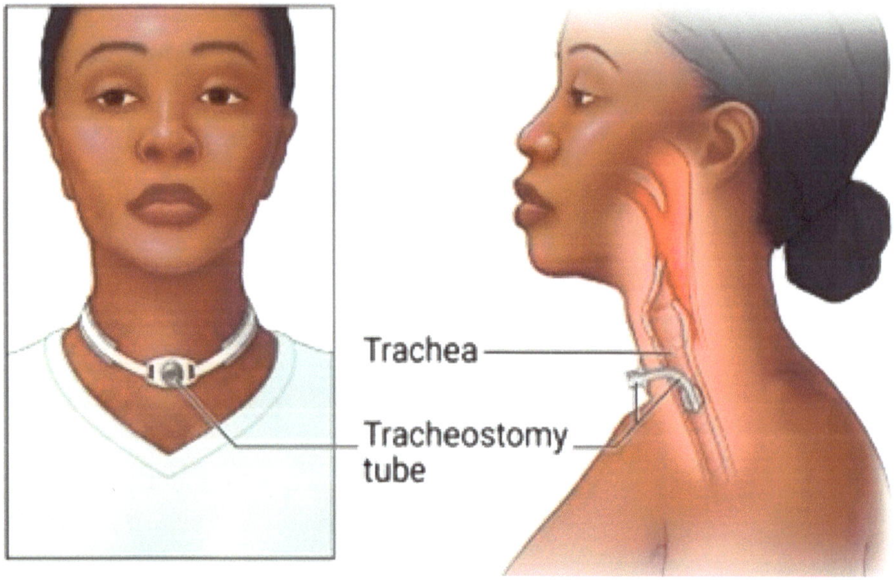

INSERTION AND REMOVAL OF FOLEY CATHETER

Steps for inserting a foley catheter:

- Open the foley catheter and lubricate generously with lubricant.
- Insert the foley catheter until you reach the "Y" of the catheter.
- Slowly inflate the balloon with the attached syringe, using the correct amount of water stated on the catheter tip in milliliters.
- Then disconnect the syringe from the foley.

How a nurse inserts a foley catheter

- Gently insert the catheter one to two inches past where the patient's urine is located.
- Using the correct amount of liquid, inflate the balloon (check the balloon size for the correct amount).
- After inflating the balloon properly, carefully pull the catheter until it is snug against the neck of the bladder.

Foley's Catheter

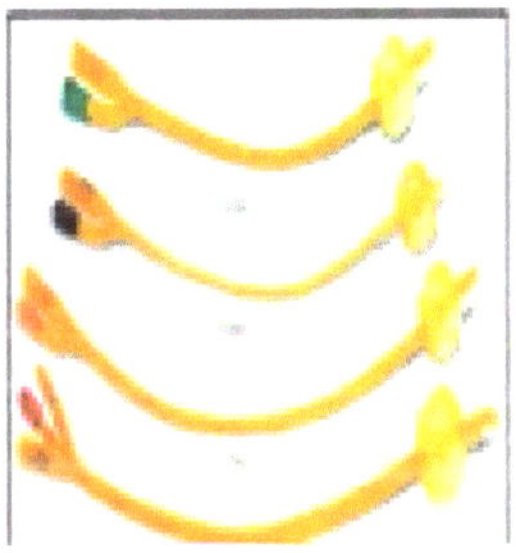

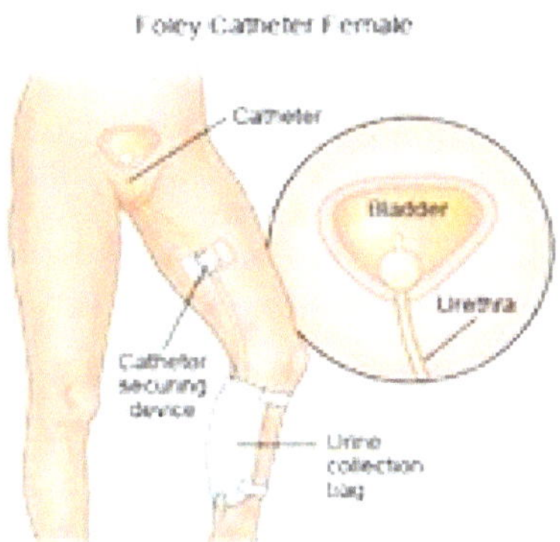

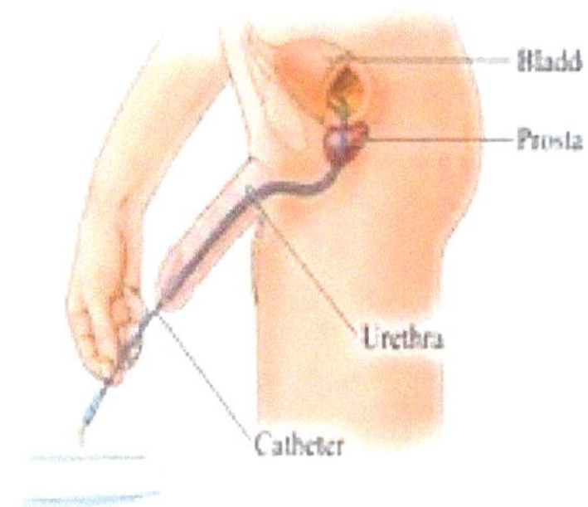

EXTERNAL FOLEY CATHETER

Pure Wick Female External Catheter from HealthyKin.com is a non-invasive wick made of soft, flexible fabric that draws urine away from the body into a collection canister. The wick should be replaced every eight to twelve hours.

Matters to consider for catheter insertion:

- Indication for catheterization
- Time and date of catheterization
- Type of catheter
- Amount of water in balloon size of the catheter
- Expiry date of product
- Any problems with the insertion
- Description of urine, color, and volume drained
- Specimen collected
- Review date.

NCLEX Practice Question:

4. The nurse assesses a client in an outpatient clinic. The client was diagnosed with osteoarthritis eighteen years ago and takes aspirin multiple times per day. Which intervention does the nurse complete first?

1 Instruct the client to take aspirin with food. Implement

2 Ask if the client has experienced gastric distress. Assessment

3 Suggest that the client take an enteric-coated aspirin. Implement
4 Determine if the client experiences tinnitus. Assessment **Correct**

Note: whenever you see a pharmacology question, you think of three things:

The intended effect of medication is to cure an ailment or to reduce symptoms.

Side effects are expected but should not be more severe than the illness itself.

Adverse effects should be monitored and managed as soon as possible. The patient should also be informed of potential side effects and their management. Regular follow-ups should be conducted to assess the effectiveness of the treatment.

5. The nurse assesses erratic electrical activity on the telemetry reading while the client is talking to the nurse on the intercom system. Which task should the nurse instruct the UAP to implement?
1 Call a code blue immediately. Implement
2 Check the client's telemetry leads. Assessment Correct.
3 Find the nurse to check on the client. Implement
4 Remove the telemetry monitor. Implement

Note: The rule of delegation says that when a nurse delegates care of a client to a staff such as LPN or UAP. The LPN or UAP who has been delegated a duty cannot re-delegate that care to another staff or LPN/UAP.

6. The client admitted to ruling out (R/O) myocardial infarction and is complaining of substernal chest pain radiating to the left arm and jaw. Which intervention should the nurse implement first?
1 Take the client's pulse, respiration, and blood pressure. Assessment
2 Call for a stat electrocardiogram and a troponin level. Implement
3 Place sublingual nitroglycerin 1/150 under the tongue. Implement Correct.
4 Notify the HCP that the client has pain. Implement

Note: The NCLEX world always thinks that you already have the order of the medication priority situation.

PHYSIOLOGICAL VS PYSCHOSOCIAL
MASLOW'S HIERARCHY OF NEEDS

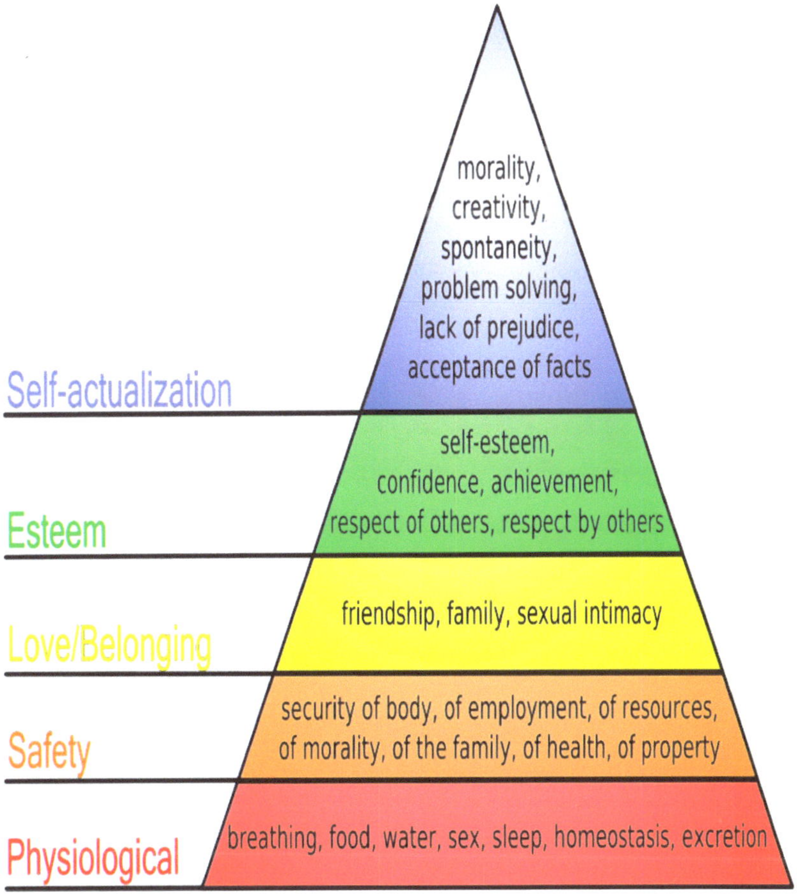

PATIENT'S PRIORITY SHOULD BE IN THE FOLLOWING ORDER:

<u>Physiology Needs</u>

Airways, e.g., air, water, food, appropriate temperature
Universal needs: food, hunger, thirst, sleep, clothing, warmth, and health
Breath, e.g., issues with breathing, hydration, nutrition, thermoregulation, or sleep is the highest priority.

Vs <u>Psychosocial Needs</u>

Pain
Education
Feelings: mental, emotional, shelter, and rest, spiritual, loneliness, grief, abuse, self-care issues
Recognition of depression, anxiety, fear, developmental problems, disability, and limitations in daily living
Lack of social and support network

HOW TO RECOGNIZE ABC QUESTION

Airway such as: gag reflex, dysphagia, swallowing
Breathing: absence of breathing sound, oxygen administration, oxygen stat, pulse oximetry, elevate HOB, use of incentive spirometry
Circulation: heart rate, PB, pulses, CPR, fluid status (fluid deficit or overload), IV fluids, TPN, central lines, bleeding/hemorrhage.

STEPS TO MASLOW'S STRATEGY

1 Do you have a mixture of physiological and psychosocial answers?
2 Eliminate all psychosocial answer choices.
3 Ask if the remainder of physiological answer choices make sense to the disease or situation.
4 Can you apply ABC if applicable?

Physiology vs Psychosocial: Whenever you have an option that contains both physical needs and psychosocial needs, you must select "physical" needs first because they are the basic needs of life. However, the bottom of the pyramid in Maslow's Hierarchy of needs is considered first as the top priority action and a physiological need is among the choices, then safety and security are the next priority before love and belonging, self-esteem, and actualization.

PRACTICE QUESTION

7. A nurse is preparing the plan of care for a client with a closed fracture of the right arm. Which problem is most appropriate for the nurse to identify?

a Risk for ineffective coping related to the inability to perform ADLs. Psychosocial
b Risk for compartment syndrome related to injured muscle tissue. Physiology
c Risk for infection related to exposed bone and tissue. Physiology
d Risk for complications related to compromised neurovascular status. Physiology/

Correct Answer: d.

8. A nurse is assigned to care for a client experiencing dystocia. When assisting with planning care, the nurse would consider the highest priority to be frequent:

a Position changes and providing comfort measures.
b Explanations to family members about what is happening to the client.
c Monitoring for changes in the physical condition of the mother and fetus.
d Reinforcement of breathing techniques learned in childbirth preparatory classes.

Correct Answer: 3.

SAAREP METHOD/STRATEGY

The mnemonic word SAAREP stands for:

S → STABLE VS UNSTABLE
A → ABC [airways, breathing, and circulation]
A → ACUTE VS CHRONIC
R → REAL PROBLEM VS POTENTIAL PROBLEM
E → EXPECTED VS UNEXPECTED
P → PHYSICAL NEEDS VS PSYCHOSOCIAL NEEDS

SAAREP METHOD/STRATEGY helps you to answer priority questions, the type of questions that indicate the need to prioritize or ask you whom to assess: first, essential, highest priority, most important, best, next, primary, immediate, vital, etc.

STABLE

- Chronic illness/slightly off lab values
- Norman lab values
- Post-Op of over > 24 hours
- Medical and other surgical
- E.g., lab value of creatinine level of 1.4; this is a stable patient

UNSTABLE

- Acute episode of sudden fever pain
- New onset/newly admitted
- Critical abnormal lab values, general anesthesia
- Unexpected signs and symptoms of any kind of sickness
- Fresh post-operative < 12 hours

Always unstable no matter what?

High fever of > 104°F (Pyrexia)

Witnessed Cardiac Arrest Patient: When you physically witness a patient collapse in front of you, then you should do the following:

- Assess for consciousness (shout the person's name)
- Call for help
- Look for CAB on the patient (circulation, airway, and breathing
- Then start compression

- **Hemorrhage: When an unstable patient is having hemorrhage,** this means internal bleeding or hemorrhage. It could be an internal vaginal hemorrhage, bladder hemorrhage, intracerebral hemorrhage (bleeding inside the brain caused by a ruptured blood vessel), hemothorax (hemorrhage inside the lungs), or cardiac tamponade (pressure on the heart that occurs when blood or fluid builds up in the space between the heart muscle and the outer covering sac of the heart).
- **Hypoglycemia –** Low glucose in the blood, e.g., a sugar level of below 70.

- **Real vs Potential Problem**
    - Real/actual problem is a problem related to an etiology manifested by signs and symptoms. For example, a patient who has a pressure ulcer due to being on bed rest.
    - Potential problems: These are problems that the patient may develop given that patient's particular circumstances and health status. For example, where there is no evidence but only a risk of the problem.
- **ABC:** Is there an answer choice where ABC is compromised? You can use Maslow's Hierarchy of Needs to answer NCLEX style questions or prioritization questions.
- **Acute has priority over chronic.** Acute is a patient condition with an abrupt onset and short duration, rapidly progressive, and in need of urgent care.
- **Chronic** is a disease lasting for months or more, and generally cannot be prevented by vaccines or cured by medication. The patient leaves with the disease.
- **Expected vs Unexpected:** Using this strategy, you must look at each option and determine what are the signs and symptoms the patients are exhibiting. Find out if they are normal or expected for the disease process. Then, if so, you do not have to see this patient first. However, if all the options include patients with expected signs and symptoms, use Maslow's Hierarchy of Needs to prioritize.

Example: a patient with type 1 diabetes mellitus with a blood glucose of 180 mg/dL (expected) while A patient with type 1 diabetes mellitus with diabetes ketoacidosis is unexpected (unexpected)

STRATEGY TO ANSWER QUESTIONS

HOW TO ANSWER QUESTIONS: There are six different types of questions The National Council of State Boards of Nursing (NCSBN) ask in the NCLEX examination. Find the below list of questions you may come across during your NCLEX.

1 Content Questions
2 Prioritization Questions
3 Delegation Questions
4 Select all that apply.
5 When to call doctor
6 Next Generation NCLEX Case Study Questions

CONTENT: The NCLEX exam consists of nursing topics. As a nursing student, you have gotten knowledge of all the topics in your nursing school. The below NCLEX key points are the area of study for the NCLEX preparation exam, which compiles all the nursing contents.

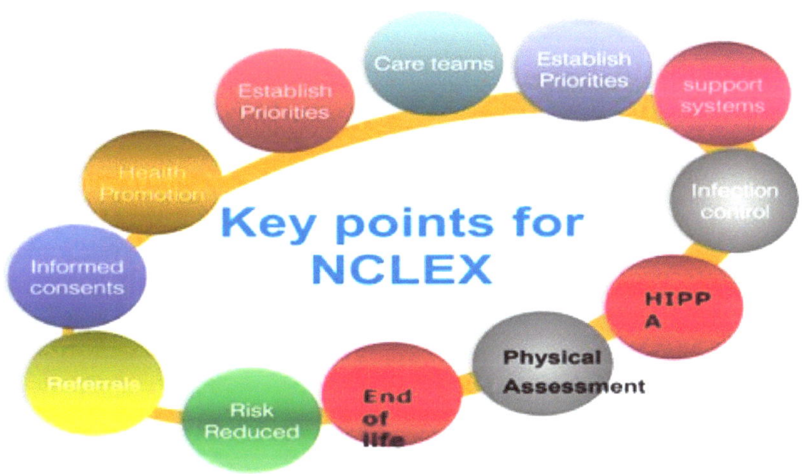

NCSBN KEY POINT FOR NCLEX

This comprises all the nursing content topics that nursing students study during their nursing school and which has the distribution of content for the NCLEX-RN/PN Test Plan. As shown below:

DISTRIBUTION OF CONTENT FOR THE NCLEX-RN® TEST PLAN

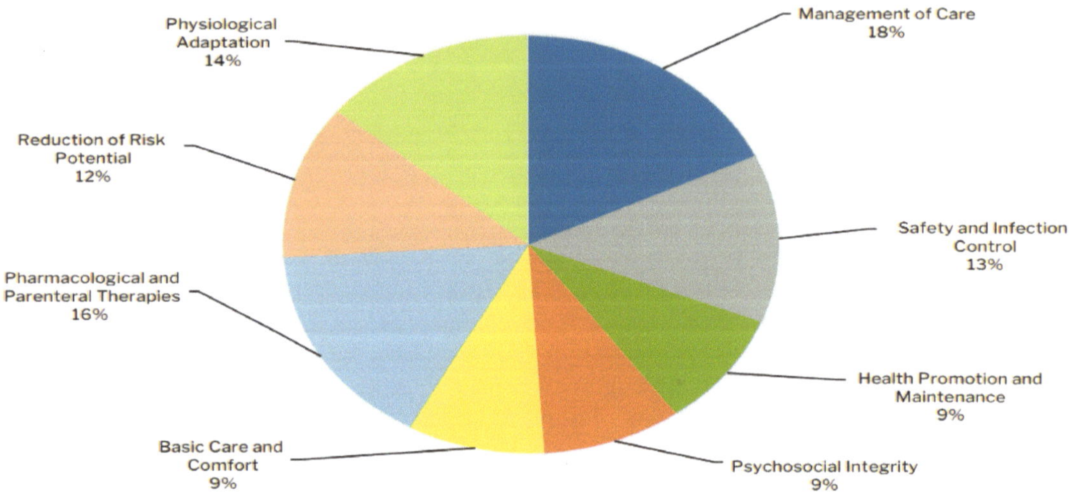

PRIORITIZATION OF CARE STRATEGY

First Level Priority Problems

- Airways
- Breathing
- Circulating and cardiac (become the first priority in cardiac arrest)
- Vital signs

Second-level Priority Problems

- Altered mental status
- Acute pain
- Untreated medical problems (e.g. hyperglycemia in a client with diabetes)
- Chronic pain

Second-level Priority Problems (continued)

- Acute elimination issues
- Abnormal laboratory results
- Risk of information and safety.

Emergency Department Triage System

Please know or memorize these priorities of care before you open the Pearson Vue door!!!

TRIAGE CATEGORY	PRIORITY	COLOR	CONDITIONS
Immediate	1	Red	Chest wounds, shock, open fractures, 2-3 degree burns
Delayed	2	Yellow	Stable abdominal wound, eye and CNS injuries
Minimal	3	Green	Minor burns, minor fractions, minor bleeding
Expectant	4	Black	Unresponsive, high spinal cord injury

Emergent (Red) Priority 1 (highest)

Life-threatening injuries and patients who need immediate care and continuous evaluation. This patient has the possibility of surviving after stabilization.

Trauma, chest pain, severe respiratory distress, cardiac arrest, limb amputation, acute neurological deficits, and chemical splashes.

Urgent (Yellow) Priority 2: Non-life-threatening injuries that are treated within one hour. This patient needs continuous evaluation every thirty to sixty minutes after treatment.

Simple fracture, asthma without respiratory distress, fever, hypertension, abnormal pain, and renal stones.

Nonurgent (Green): Priority 3:

This is given to patients with local injuries who do not have immediate complications and who can wait several hours for medical treatment; these clients require an evaluation every one to two hours after treatment.

Minor lacerations, sprains, and cold symptoms.

PRACTICE QUESTION

The nurse is preparing to enter a disaster scene to assist with triaging victims. What assessment priorities should the nurse adhere to? **Select all that apply.**

1. The nurse requires disaster certification before performing triage during a disaster.
2. The nurse should consider the age of a victim before allocating any resources.
3. The nurse must consult a qualified healthcare provider prior to making client resource decisions.
4. The nurse should assess clients by considering their airways, breathing, circulation, and neurological function. Correct!
5. The nurse should allocate resources to those victims with the strongest probability of survival. Correct!

Answer: 4 and 5

RATIONALE

The goal of disaster triage is to use resources for clients with the strongest probability of survival. Age is not a consideration when allocating treatment resources, and the nurse does not need to consult a physician prior to making decisions about allocating resources. Furthermore, a nurse does not need special training to assist in a disaster. However, there are certifications available for nurses who are interested. Finally, the nurse will make decisions based on a client's airway, breathing, circulation, and neurological function.

DELEGATION, ASSIGNMENT, AND SUPERVISION STRATEGY

- **DELEGATION:** The definition of delegation alone offers some important clues to nursing practice and to the composition of an effective patient care team. The person who makes the decision to ask a person to do something (a task or assignment) must know that the chosen person is competent to perform that task. RNs select tasks, given their knowledge of the individual patient's condition and that circumstance because of the nurse's preparation, knowledge, and skill. The RN chooses to render judgments of this kind and stands by the choices made. According to licensure and statute, the nurse is obligated to delegate based on the unique situation, patients, and personnel involved, and to provide ongoing follow-up.
- **ASSIGNMENT:** The definition of assignment is described as what a person is directed to do. Also, assignment is a work plan; the nurse "assigns" or distributes work and "delegates" nursing care as she or he works through others.
- **SUPERVISION** is defined by NCSBN as "the provision of guidance and direction, oversight, evaluation and follow up by the licensed nurse for the accomplishment of a nursing task delegated to nursing assistive personnel" (NCSBN, 2005, p 194).
- The act of delegation is just the beginning of the RN's responsibility. As for the accountability of the delegates (or persons given the task duty), these individuals are accountable for "[accepting] the delegation and for their own actions in carrying out the act" (NCSBN, 1995, p 3).

MORE SIMPLIFIED DEFINITION OF DELEGATION STRATEGY

Delegation means assigning responsibility for a task on your to-do list to someone else, so you can focus on something more pressing that requires your expertise.

For all tasks delegated by the nurse to other staff, the delegating nurse must take full responsibility/accountability for the task delegated.

The six rights of the delegation are included:

The right tasks

Right circumstances

Right person

Right direction/communication

Right supervision/evaluation

Right documentation

There are two main key components in successfully answering questions on delegation. Ensure to memorize the general roles, responsibilities, and scopes, and analyze the delegation principles.

What is the role of a Registered Nurse (RN)

What is the role of a Licensed Practical Nurse (LPN) and

What is the role of a Certified Nurse Assistance (CNA)

To answer the correct option, do remember that the NCLEX® is textbook-based and written to test the student's (text-taker's) knowledge of general delegation principles.

SCOPE OF PRACTICE:

Registered Nurse

Admission and discharge of patient and refer patient to other providers
Responsible for assessment and planning of care
Initiating teaching
Initial care of the patient after the surgical operation
Delegate appropriate tasks to both LPN/LVNs and UAPs
Initiate and administer blood to a patient
Administration of high-risk medications intravenously and via IV push
Independently monitor and titrate medications
Performs any tasks that may be performed by LPN or LVNs and UAPs

Licensed Practical Nurse (LPN) scope of practice

LPN are also nurses
Medication administration (routine and stable clients)
Do more than UAP
Sterile procedures
Administer urine catheter
Ostomy care
Phlebotomy
Enteral feeding
Assist the registered nurse (RN) with collecting data and monitoring patient findings
Administer a nasogastric (NG) tube feeding
Perform wound dressing changes
Do tracheostomy care
Reinforce an RN's patient education, but do not perform independent patient education or assessments
Perform suctioning
Specific or focus assessment (lung sounds, bowel sounds, neurovascular checks)
Reinforcing education
Changing dressings (wound care)
Skin care
Giving enema
Helping with activities of daily living

Unlicensed Assistive Personnel (UAP) is the same as CNA, Nursing Assistive Personnel (NAP), nursing assistants, nurse aides, orderlies, assistance, and attendants.

Collect observational data
Take vital signs (routine and stable clients)

Bedside care
Encourage hydration
Bathing
Positioning
Feeding
Linen change
Monitor and record intake and output
Weighting clients
Gathering equipment
Helping with activities of daily living
Ambulate stable patient

DELEGATION GUIDELINES

The registered nurse delegates the most critical client or patient to the most qualified or experienced nurse.
Do not delegate the care of unstable patients to LPN and UAP.
Remember to discharge the most stable patient.
Admit the most unstable person in the intensive care unit (ICU).
The registered nurse takes responsibility for all tasks delegated.
Registered nurse is responsible for assessment and planning of care, initiating teaching, and administering medications intravenously (IV).
The registered nurse ensures continuity of care while delegating patient care.
Principles for the Implementation of Prioritization, Delegation, and Assignment
The RN should have a patient purpose and preferred outcome in mind.
The RN should refer to the applicable state nursing practice statute and rules and the facility's job descriptions for current information about the roles and responsibilities of RNs, LPNs/LVNs, and UAPs.
The student nurses, novices, float nurses, and other infrequent workers will also require varying levels of supervision, guidance, or support.
The RN is accountable for nursing judgment decisions and for ongoing supervision of any care that is delegated or assigned.
Registered nurse must be knowledgeable about patients, their conditions, as well as team members' skills and competencies. Prioritization, delegation, and assignment are all part of their responsibilities.

ROLE TRANSITIONING TO LEADERSHIP/MANAGEMENT

Identify ways a nurse can transition to a leadership role: As a nurse leader, you cannot avoid the added responsibilities and demands, but without time management skills, it will be difficult to transition into your leadership role. A great nurse leader needs to properly manage conflicts in the workplace and should have the ability to recognize and address problems quickly.
Effective communication: It is important that nurses have effective communication, both verbal and non-verbal, as well as listening skills. A great nurse leader needs to clearly communicate his or her ideas, visions, goals, and expectations to staff nurses and others as well as understand what other people are communicating.

CRITICAL THINKING: A great nurse leader needs to be able to think objectively and critically as well as utilize critical thinking ability at every level. Critical thinking is the utmost to a leader's success, especially in today's complex healthcare environment. Having an optimistic attitude is also important as this will help to motivate other staff nurses in a positive way.

TIME MANAGEMENT: A great nurse leader needs to effectively manage time and fulfill his or her tasks and obligations. As a nurse leader, you cannot avoid the added responsibilities and demands, but without time management skills, it will be difficult to transition into your leadership role.

CONFLICT MANAGEMENT: A great nurse leader needs to properly manage conflicts in the workplace. You should have the ability to recognize and address problems quickly. Stress disappears, staff feels more motivated, and the workplace becomes a much better place to work because of conflict management.

ACTIVITY COMPLETION
All tasks are evaluated on completion.
Use the scope of practice to evaluate staff members, training, and experience.
Evaluate the effectiveness of staff time management.

Case Management:
Referrals to appropriate HCP resources available to assist the client with maintaining or achieving independence and assess the client's need for materials and equipment (e.g., oxygen, suction machine, wound care supplies)
Provide cost-effective care. Plan individualized care for the client based on need (e.g., client diagnosis, self-care ability)
Prescribed treatments. Provide client with information on discharge procedures for home, hospice, or community settings. Use care maps and or clinical pathway to initiate, evaluate, and update the plan of care.

EMERGENCY/TRAUMA ASSESSMENT

Management of Trauma Patients

Primary and secondary methods of caring for the emergency/trauma patient, using mnemonic: **Primary-ABCDE, and Secondary-FGHI.**

Primary survey is a standardized way of performing the initial assessment of all trauma patients and should be done the same every single time and case, so you do not miss out on anything. The major goal of the primary survey is as follows: first, to identify life threats quickly, and second, to provide stability when life threats are identified.

A – AIRWAYS: Clear airway, stabilize cervical spine injury, high C-spine injury will impair respiratory drive (C3-C5)

B – Breathing: Give oxygen, prepare to intubate, check tension pneumothorax (treat with needle decompression), open pneumothorax (treat with occlusive dressing), flail chest (treat with supportive (intubate, ventilate)), massive hemothorax (treat with tube thoracostomy, i.e. A procedure in which fluid, blood, or air are drained from the lung's surrounding area)

C – Circulating: Check for pulse and heart rate, control bleeding/external bleeding, then look for: the color of skin, LOC (level of consciousness), capillary refill, and feel peripheral pulse strength.

D – Disability: Check for level of consciousness and assess using the Glasgow coma scale; also use abbreviations such as the AVE Pugh scale which is alert, verbal pain, or unresponsive. This means the patient is alert and normal, they respond only to verbal stimuli, they respond only to painful stimuli, or they are completely unresponsive.

E – Exposure: Remove clothing and prevent heat loss.

SECONDARY SURVEY: This is done when normal vital signs are present.

F – Full set of vital signs/focused interventions: monitor ECG, place tube and drains

G – Give comfort: assess and treat pain

H – Head-to-toe assessment: history: use SAMPLE, which stands for:

S - signs and symptoms

A - allergies

M - medications

P- Past medical/health history

Secondary Survey (continued)

L - Last Meal - help us to know how much meal can be in the patient's stomach before surgery or treatment

E - Events preceding, the environment

I – Inspect posterior: log roll and palpate the patient.

PRACTICE QUESTION

1.The nurse is working on an orthopedic floor. Which client should the nurse assess first after the change of shift report?

a The eighty-six-year-old female with a fractured right femoral neck in Buck's traction.

b The sixty-six-year-old female with a left total knee replacement has confusion.

c The eighty-nine-year-old male patient right total hip replacement with an abduction pillow.

d The fifty-year-old postop client with a continuous (CPM) device.

Correct Answer: b

2. The home health nurse must see the following clients. Which client the nurse should assess first?

a The client is a post-op from an open cholecystectomy and has green drainage coming from the T-tube. Chronic/Expected

b The client was diagnosed with congestive heart failure and complains of shortness of breath while fixing meals. **Chronic/Expected**

c The client was diagnosed with AIDS dementia whose family called and reported that the client is vomiting coffee ground stuff. **Chronic/Airways (Unstable ABC)**

d The client diagnosed with end-stage liver failure has gained three pounds and is not able to wear house shoes. **Chronic/Expected**

Correct Answer: c

3. A nurse is assigned to care for four clients. When planning client rounds, which client would the nurse check first?

1 A client on a ventilation Correct

2 A client in skeletal traction

3 A postoperative client preparing for discharge

4 A client admitted on the previous shift has a diagnosis of gastroenteritis

Correct answer 1

Rationale: Use the ABC (airways, breathing, and circulation) to answer the question. The word "ventilation" is air circulation. The circulation and exchange of gases in the lungs is basic to respiration. So the nurse will check this client's ventilation status first.

The employed in an emergency department is assigned to triage clients coming to the emergency department for treatment on the evening shift. The nurse should assign priority to which client?

1 A client complaining of muscle aches, a headache, and a history of seizures

2 A client who twisted her ankle when rollerblading and is requesting medication for pain

3 A client with a minor laceration on the index finger sustained while cutting an eggplant

4 A client with chest pain states that he just ate pizza that was made with a very spicy sauce. correct
Correct answer 4.
Rationale: Use ABC (airway, breathing, circulation) to direct you to the correct option. A client experiencing chest pain is always classified as Priority 1 until MI has been ruled out.

4. The nurse is evaluating the response to the plan of care for a client who abuses alcohol. Which of the following statements by the client would indicate that the client's treatment regimen has been effective? **Select all that apply.**
1. "I will be able to stop drinking alcohol if my spouse can prevent me from experiencing the financial stress we have experienced in the past."
2. "I would like to obtain a referral to a dietitian in order to learn about what food I should eat to maintain a more balanced diet." Correct
3. "I can drink small amounts of alcohol at family celebrations and important religious ceremonies."
4. "I plan to telephone my Alcoholics Anonymous (AA) sponsor if I feel the need to drink alcohol." Correct
5. "I understand that personal willpower can prevent me from drinking alcohol again." Correct
Correct answer 2,4, and 5.
Rationale: option 2, 4and 5 are correct because the patient who abuses alcohol and attend the Al-Anon meeting should have a positive response in other to stop drinking alcohol.

5.The nurse provides care to a newly diagnosed patient with schizophrenia who is prescribed chlorpromazine 25 mg PO bid. Which patient statement indicates a correct understanding of taking the medication? **(Select all that apply.)**
a I'll brush my teeth three times a day. **Correct**
b It may take four to six weeks for my medication to start working. **Correct**
c I may have a glass of wine each night because it is good for the heart.
d I can drive myself to work on Monday.
e I must get blood levels regularly for a couple of months. **Correct**
f I will not worry about pink urine.
Correct: a, b, & e.

HEALTHCARE TEAM COMMUNICATION

REPORT: A nurse should always give a factual, accurate, current, complete, organized, and confidential report to the physician about the status of the patient. The report should include the following:
SBAR TECHNIQUE: S=subject B=background A=assessment R=recommendation
Background information
Subjective data
Objection data

Any change in the patient's status
Nursing diagnosis
Treatment and procedures
Medication administration, client teaching, discharge planning, family information
The patient's response to treatments and procedures
The patient's priority needs

SELECT ALL THAT APPLY STRATEGY

KNOWING THE QUESTIONS:

It is very important to familiarize yourself with answering this type of question as it requires you to move the answers into the appropriate order depending on the type of question. Some questions ask a situational approach in accordance with their priority (example: who would you assess first from the following clients?), application of nursing process (ADPIE), nursing procedures (example removing personal protective equipment), and nursing diagnosis (actual, wellness, and risk).
"Select all that applies" questions show how you're doing on the NCLEX. A common myth about Select All That Applies (SATA) questions is that if you get a lot of them on your test, you're passing. Answer the SATA questions in a manner of true or false statements and always select two or more answers.
Important Reminder: Most test-takers have a mental pattern in answering this type of question. They think they need to add another answer because the previously selected options are not enough. Select only the options that are the perfect fit for the question.
Know When to Call the Doctor: Before choosing to notify the physician, you must first ask yourself some questions, such as:

Did I assess the client, e.g. vital signs?
Is there any intervention I need to provide for the patient?
Is it outside the scope of the duty of a registered nurse (RN)?
Does the client have an immediate need but require the action of a physician?

The nurse is teaching a client who is scheduled for a total hip arthroplasty via a posterior approach. Which of the following information should the nurse include? **Select all that apply.**

1 "The type of prosthesis used is based on the muscle strength and joint function of your upper extremities."
2 "Do not bend the affected hip more than 90 degrees after surgery." **Correct**
3 "Skin preparation and cleansing is mandatory before surgery." **Correct**
4 "Use an elevated toilet seat for at least six weeks after surgery." **Correct**
5 "You can resume sexual intercourse after surgery if your partner is in a dependent position."

Correct answer: 3, 4, 5

The nurse is assessing a client with suspected gout. Which of the following findings would support a diagnosis of gout? Select all that apply.
1. Elevated serum uric acid level Correct
2. A swollen, red joint Correct
3. Reports of moderate fatigue
4. Distal extremities cool to touch
5. Pain associated with movement of the affected extremity Correct
6. Intolerance of dairy products Correct
Correct answer: 1, 2, 5, 6

The nurse is planning to care for a client who has expressive aphasia after a left-sided stroke. Which of the following statements by the client's spouse would indicate a correct understanding of the client's communication abilities and interaction needs? Select all that apply.
1. "My spouse's response of 'fine' when asked how the day has been may or may not be what my spouse meant to communicate." Correct
2. "I can anticipate what my spouse wants to say, so I complete my spouse's sentences to make communication quicker."
3. "I will purchase a picture board to help my spouse express common needs, thoughts, and feelings that are difficult to communicate." Correct
4. "My spouse's angry response when we have a conversation makes me hesitant to try further communication."
5. "I have arranged for my spouse to meet with a speech therapist twice each week to improve communication skills." Correct
Correct answer: 1, 3, 5

The nurse is planning care for a client with moderate Alzheimer's disease (AD). Which of the following interventions should the nurse include in the client's plan of care? Select all that apply.
1. Establish a daily routine for the client.
2. Assist the client to void every two hours.
3. Introduce yourself upon interacting with the client.
4. Display a clock and calendar in the client's room.
5. Keep the client's television on during the day to distract the client.
Correct answer: 1, 2, 3, 4

The nurse is teaching a client who is scheduled for a paracentesis in six hours. Which of the following information should the nurse include? Select all that apply.
1. "You should maintain a supine position for the procedure."
2. "Your weight will be obtained before and after the procedure."
3. "You will be transported to the radiology department for the procedure."
4. "Your bladder will need to be emptied prior to the procedure."
5. "You will need to avoid eating or drinking for two hours prior to the procedure."
Correct answer: 1, 2, 4

The nurse is planning care for a client who had a stroke and has unilateral neglect. Which of the following interventions should the nurse include in the client's plan of care? Select all that apply.
1. Teach the client to scan the environment.
2. Approach the client on the client's unaffected side.
3. Instruct the client to dress the unaffected side first.
4. Initiate the conversation by touching the client's affected shoulder.
5. Rearrange the environment to compensate for the client's visual deficits.
Correct answer: 1, 2, 5

INFECTION CONTROL

STANDARD PRECAUTION: Dress for what you see. This is practiced for all patients in any setting, regardless of the diagnosis or the assumed infectiousness.

Promote hand hygiene and the use of gloves, masks, eye protection, foot protection, and gowns, when applicable, especially during patient contact. Also, these precautions apply to blood, all body fluids, secretions, and excretions, regardless of whether they contain blood, nonintact skin, or mucous membrane.

INTERVENTIONS

All blood and body fluids from all patients should be handled as if they were contaminated.

Hand hygiene/hand washing with soap and water, or an alcohol-based hand rub is necessary to decontaminate the hands before having direct contact with a patient.

Hands must be washed with soap and water between contact with a patient after contact with blood, body fluids, secretions, or excretions, and after contact with equipment and immediately after removal of gloves.

Masks, eye protection, or face shields are worn if patient care activities may generate splashes or sprays of blood or body fluid.

All contaminated linens are placed in leakproof bags and handled to prevent skin and mucous membrane exposure.

PERSONAL PROTECTIVE EQUIPMENT (PPE)

Donning: putting on PPE

Put on PPE before entering the client's room.

Do not touch your face while wearing PPE.

Avoid touching areas in the client's room.

STAFF WEAR PPE

Gown

Mask or respirator

Goggles or face shield

Gloves

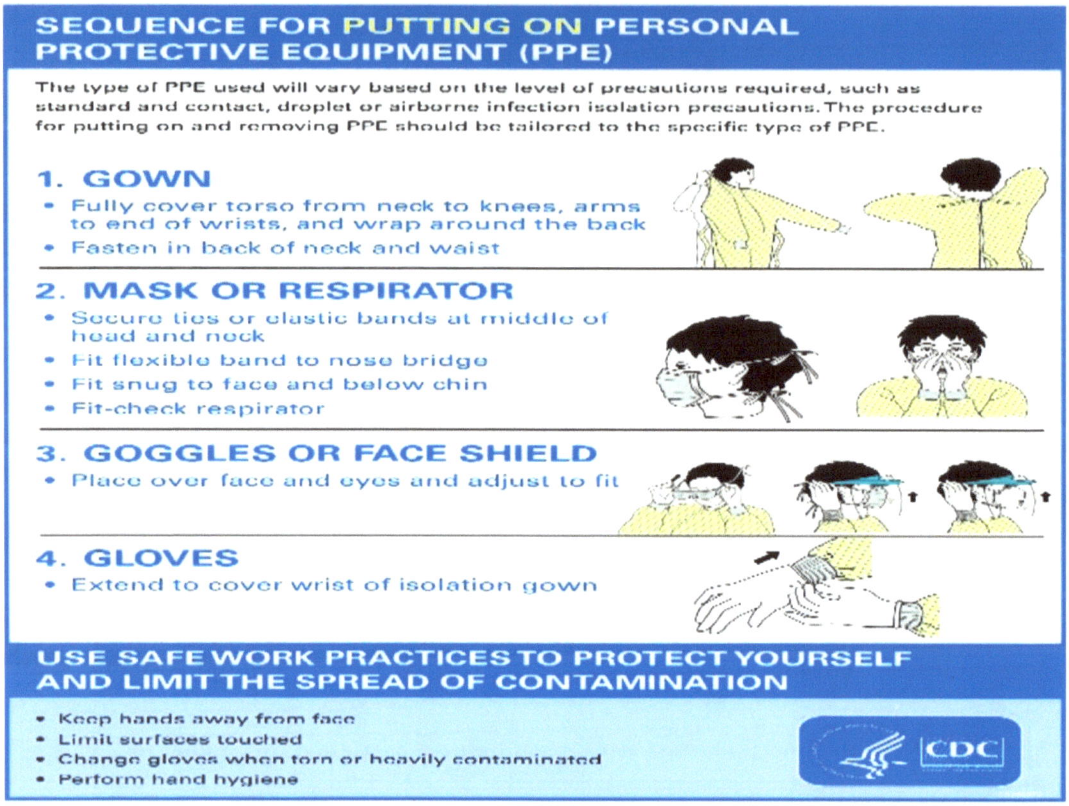

DOFFING: REMOVING PPE

Remove PPE at the patient's doorway or outside the room.

If hands become soiled while removing PPE, stop and perform hand hygiene. Then, continue with PPE removal:

Gloves

Goggles/face shield

Gown

Mask/respirator

Hand hygiene

DOFFING: REMOVING PPE

Gown and gloves

Goggle or face shield

Masks or respirators

Wash hands or use as alcohol-based hand sanitizer

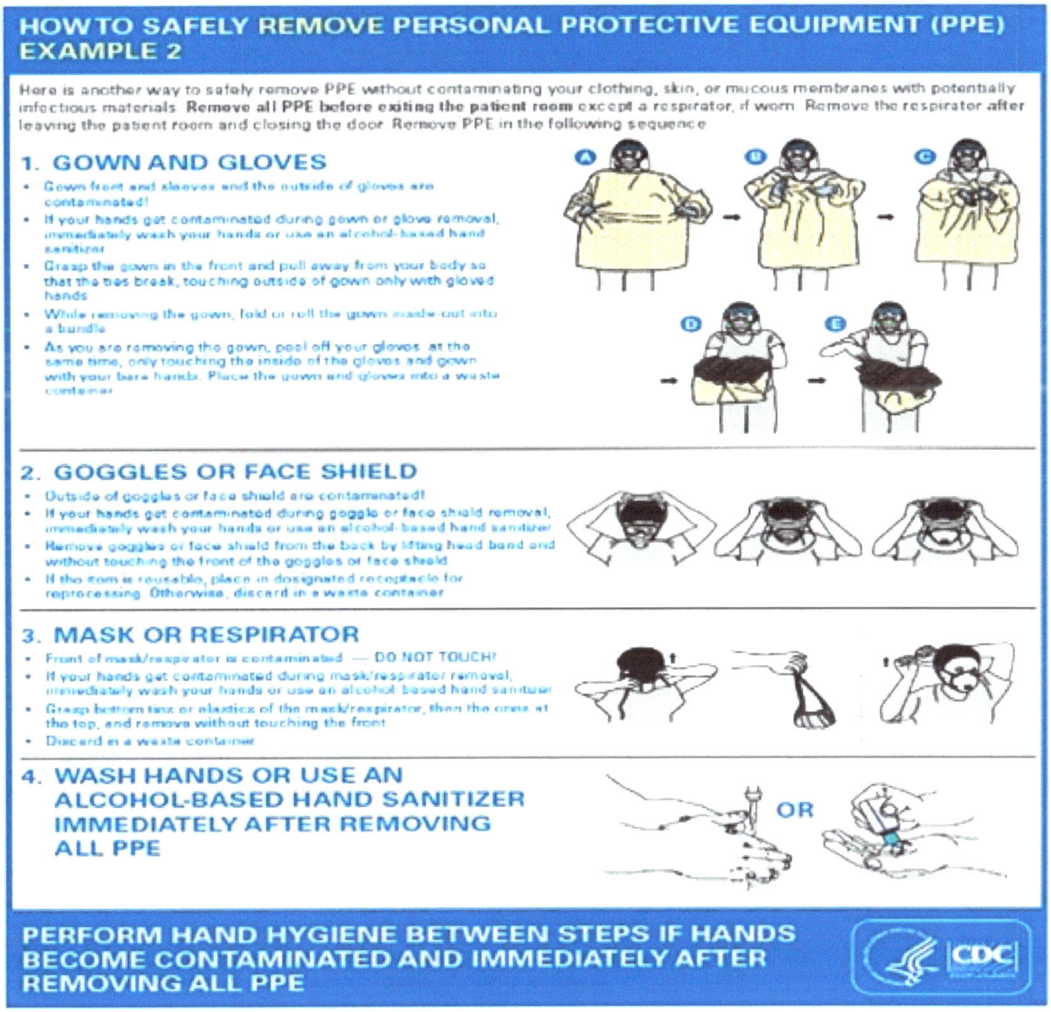

HOSPITAL-ASSOCIATED INFECTIONS

HAI - Hospital-associated infection

CAUTI - Catheter-associated urinary tract infection

SSI - Surgical site infection

CLABSI - Central line-associated blood infection

VAP – Ventilator-associated pneumonia

*Note: Meticulous hand hygiene practices and the use of chlorhexidine solution helps in preventing HAIs.

CHAIN OF INFECTION

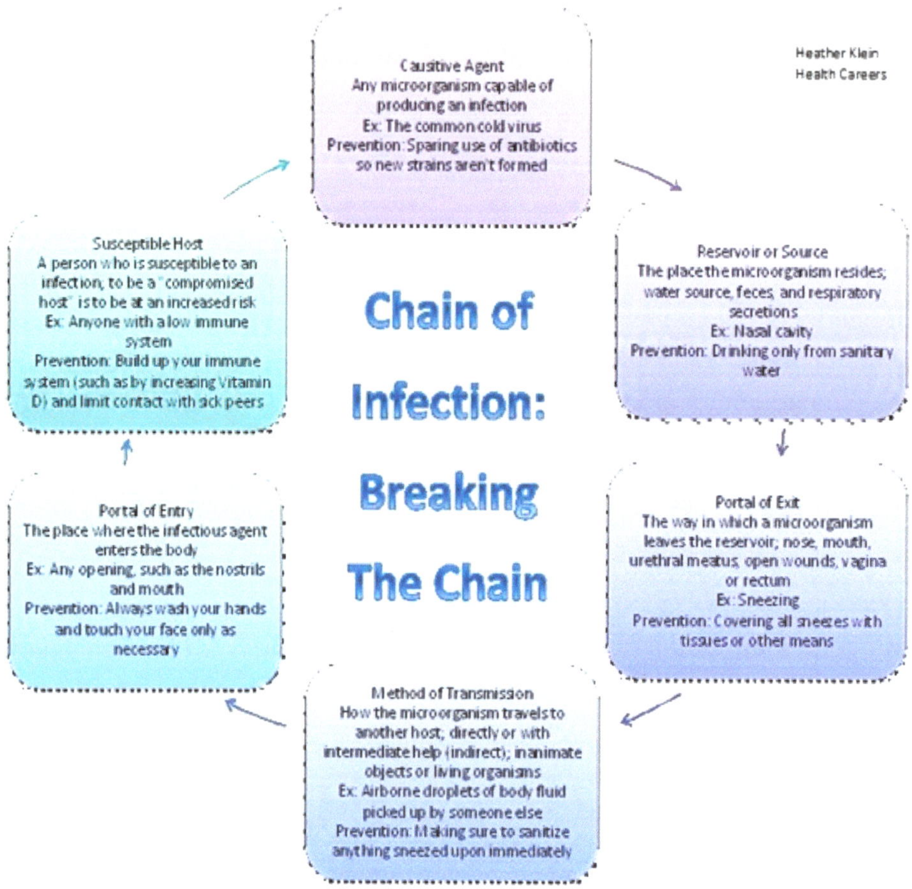

The Infectious Disease Model On Cross Transmission Of Microbes [Germs] Or...

How Microbes Move around

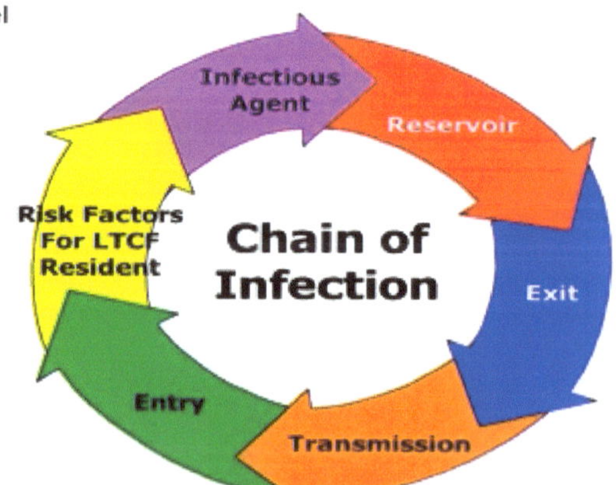

LTCF = long term care facility

TRANSMISSION-BASED PRECAUTIONS

AIRBORNE

Single room under negative pressure

The door remains closed.

Healthcare workers wear a respiratory mask (N95 or higher level) and gloves.

Think "MTV"

M = Measles

T = Tuberculosis

V = Varicella (chickenpox) and disseminated herpes-zoster (shingles)

Note: Airborne is no longer needed when all lesions have crusted over.

DROPLET PRECAUTION

A private room or a patient whose body culture contains the same organism

Wear a surgical mask.

Place a mask on the patient whenever they leave the room.

Think of Spiderman (mnemonic)

Sepsis

Scarlet fever

Streptococcal pharyngitis

Parvovirus B19

Pneumonia

Pertussis

Influenza

Diphtheria (pharyngeal)

Epiglottitis

Rubella

Mumps

Meningitis

Mycoplasma or meningeal pneumonia

Adenovirus

PPE: gloves and masks

Note: Include GOWN if there are splashes of fluid and blood, skin rashes with blisters, and emesis (vomiting).

CONTACT PRECAUTIONS

Private room or cohort client

Use gloves and a gown whenever entering the patient's room.

Colonization or infection with a multidrug-resistant organism

Enteric infections (clostridium difficile)

Respiratory infections (RSV influenza)

Wound and skin infections (cutaneous diphtheria, herpes simples, impetigo, pediculosis, scabies, staphylococci, and varicella-zoster)
Eye infections (conjunctivitis)

Think MRS. WEE

M = Multidrug-resistant organism
R = Respiratory infection
S = Skin infections
W = wound infection
E = Enteric infection (clostridium difficile)
E = Eye infection (conjunctivitis)

SKIN INFECTIONS: Think VCHIPS (MNEMONIC)

V = Varicella-zoster
C = Cutaneous diphtheria
H = Herpes simplex
I = Impetigo
P = Pediculosis
S = Scabies

PPE: gloves and gown

HEALTH PROMOTION AND MAINTENANCE

Health Screening and Health Promotion Review

US HEALTH STATISTICS

Mortality Statistics

Leading cause of death (all ages/genders):

Heart disease (or diseases of the heart)

Cancer (or malignant neoplasms)

Chronic lower respiratory diseases (i.e., chronic obstructive pulmonary disease [COPD])

Cancer Mortality

Leading cause of cancer death:

Lung cancer

Leading causes of cancer deaths in men:

Lung cancer

Prostate cancer

Colorectal cancer

Leading causes of cancer deaths in women:

Lung cancer

Breast cancer

Colorectal cancer

Leading Causes of Death in Adolescents

Death rate for teen males is higher than for females:

Accidents/unintentional injuries (39.5%): The most common cause is motor vehicle crashes (risk is highest from 16 to 19 years of age)

Suicide (16.8%): Watch teens for signs of depression, excess stress, and suicidal behavior; open communication between the adolescent and the parents/caregivers (or persons they trust) is extremely important in preventing teenage suicide.

Death rate for teen males is higher than for females:

Homicide (14.3%): Nonfatal and fatal violence is much higher among young people compared to any other age group.

Leading Cause of Mortality by Age Group:

Birth to 12 months: congenital malformations (20.3%)

Ages 1 to 44 years: unintentional injuries (23.2 %)

Ages 45 to 64 years: cancer (30.9%)

Ages 65 and older: heart disease (25.6%)

Life Expectancy

Life expectancy for the US population in 2020 was 77.0 years, a decrease of 1.8 years from 2019. National Center for Health Statistics. Mortality in the United States, 2020. https://www.cdc.gov/nchs/data/databriefs/db427.pdf

Data from the National Vital Statistics System

Age-specific death rates increased from 2019 to 2020 for each age group fifteen years and over.

Nine of the ten leading causes of death in 2020 remained the same as in 2019, although five causes switched rank; heart disease and cancer remained the top two leading causes, and COVID-19 became the third leading cause of death in 2020.

The infant mortality rate decreased by 2.9% in 2020 from 2019 to a record low of 541.9 infant deaths per 100,000 live births.

DISEASE AND DEATH PREVENTION

Primary Prevention (Prevention of Disease/Injury)

Individual actions (healthy individuals): eat a nutritious diet, exercise, use seatbelts, and helmets.

Gun safety: use safety locks for guns; keep guns out of reach of children/teens.

National programs: Federal health promotion/disease-prevention programs include immunizations, Occupational Safety and

Health Administration (OSHA)'s job safety laws, and

Environmental Protection Agency (EPA) laws.

Programs promote a healthy lifestyle for youth (healthy diet, exercise, etc.)

Building a youth center in an urban high-crime area or a Habitat for Humanity (shelter)

Aspirin prophylaxis is the primary prevention of CVD and colon cancer in adults aged 50 to 59 years who have a 10% risk or higher.

Secondary Prevention (Early Detection of a Disease to Minimize Bodily Damage)

Screening tests (pap smears, mammograms, CBC for anemia, etc.)

Screening for depression (interviewing a patient about feelings of sadness, hopelessness)

Screening for sexually transmitted infections (STIs; asking about sexual history, partners, signs, and symptoms)

Screening for alcohol abuse (interviewing a patient using the CAGE questionnaire)

Testing for hepatitis C virus infection in a person with risk factors

Having a person with a history of MI, TIA, or stroke take an aspirin or statin daily (to prevent a future stroke or MI).

Tertiary Prevention (Prevention of Disease Progression)

Rehabilitation, support groups, education on equipment

Support groups: Alcoholics Anonymous (AA), breast cancer support groups, HIV support groups
Education for patients with the pre-existing disease (i.e., diabetes, hypertension): avoidance of drug interactions, proper use of wheelchair or medical equipment, others
Rehabilitation: cardiac rehabilitation, physical therapy (PT), occupational therapy (OT)
Treatment of a person with hepatitis C virus infection
Treatment of a person who has already had a heart attack with daily aspirin (to prevent another heart attack)

US PREVENTIVE SERVICES TASK FORCE

Aspirin Use to Prevent Cardiovascular Disease and Colorectal Cancer (April 2016)

Age fifty to fifty-nine years with equal or more than 10% risk (ten-year cardiovascular disease risk)
Initiate low-dose aspirin use for primary prevention of cardiovascular and colorectal cancer (in patients who are not at increased risk for bleeding) with a life expectancy of at least ten years and who are willing to take low-dose aspirin daily for at least ten years.

Breast Cancer (January 2016)

Baseline mammogram: Start at age fifty years and repeat every two years until the age of seventy-four years
Age seventy-five years or older: insufficient evidence for a routine mammogram
Does not apply to women with known genetic mutations (BRCA1 or BRCA2), familial breast cancer, history of chest radiation at a young age, or previously diagnosed with high-risk breast lesions who may benefit from starting screening in their forties.
NOTE: Age forty to forty-nine years (individualized based on risk factors, if done).
The American Cancer Society recommends starting routine screening at the age of forty years.

CERVICAL CANCER SCREENING

The most common type of cancer in women is cervical cancer. Cervical cancer can be detected early and treated more effectively with regular screening tests. A Pap test and HPV test are important screening tests. A cervical cancer screening should be conducted every three to five years for women. In addition to preventing cervical cancer, vaccines are also effective. There is a potential for life-saving benefits from regular screenings and vaccinations.

The nurse informed the parents of an 11-year-old female patient about their doctor's appointment for the HPV vaccine. What is this vaccine for?

1) It's for the prevention of breast cancer
2) this vaccine helps reduce leukemia
3) this vaccine helps reduce lung cancer
4) Help prevent cervical cancer. Correct

Rationale: As a preventative measure, the CDC recommends HPV vaccination between the ages of 11 and 12 (or as early as age 9 if you are not vaccinated already), and up to the age of 26 if you have not already had it.

CAUSES OF CARDIAC ARREST

There are several causes of cardiac arrest, including an electrical malfunction in the heart and a loss of blood flow to the brain. A variety of factors can contribute to this, including heart attacks, electrolyte imbalances, and certain medications. Some lifestyle choices, medical conditions, and trauma can also lead to these conditions. A cardiac arrest can be prevented by early detection and treatment.

5 Hs and Ts of Cardiac Arrest

1 Hypoglycemia – medical emergency – low blood sugar level in the body (>70 mg/dL)
2 Hypothermia – medical emergency – low body temperature (95 F (35 C))
3 Hypovolemia - Low extracellular fluid volume. Caused by loss of bodily fluids or blood.
4 Hypoxia, hydrogen ion (acidosis) - The body receives insufficient oxygen leading to metabolic acidosis, as ATP synthesis increases through anaerobic metabolic processes, hydrogen ions increase, and pH decreases.
5 Hypokalemia – low potassium in the body Alcohol abuse (excessive).

Chronic kidney disease.

- Diabetic ketoacidosis (in which the body has elevated levels of blood acids called ketones)
- Diarrhea.
- Diuretics (water retention relievers).
- Excessive laxative use.
- Excessive sweating.
- Folic acid deficiency.
- or hyperkalemia.- high potassium in the body.
- Hyperkalemia is caused by the following factors:
- Diseases of the kidneys.
- Diabetic disease,
- Using chemotherapy,
- An extremely traumatic event.
- Rhabdomyolysis and crush injuries.

Injuries that severely damage or burn the blood cells can cause dehydration (lack of enough water and other fluids to function normally). Overuse of potassium supplements. Diabetes type 1.

5 Ts of Cardiac Arrest

Toxins (overdoses)

Tamponade

Thrombosis

Tension Pneumothorax

Trauma

Toxins (overdoses)

Overdose toxicity refers to serious, often harmful, and sometimes fatal toxic reactions to an accidental overdose of a drug (because of an error on the part of the doctor, pharmacist, or person taking the drug) or to an intentional overdose (homicide or suicide).

INITIAL SYMPTOMS	ACUTE SYMPTOMS
• Nausea	• Seizures
• Vomiting	• Failing, Respiration (difficulty breathing)
• Acute diarrhea	• Irregular Heartbeat
• Drowsiness	• Unconsciousness or deep sleep you can't wake them from, even if they are snoring it could be drug-related
• Dizziness	• gurgling
• Confusion	• Turning blue
• Pale, cool or clammy skin	

Causes of Overdose: Overdoses can be caused by misusing prescription drugs, using illegal drugs, or taking a combination of drugs. This can lead to physical and psychological distress, long-term health problems, and in some cases, even death. It is important to be aware of the risks associated with drug use and to take steps to protect your health. Talk to your doctor about any prescription drugs you are taking and be sure to follow the directions. Never mix drugs or take more than the recommended dose.

CARDIAC TAMPONADE

Cardiac tamponade has the following symptoms:

- Anxiety and restlessness
- Low blood pressure
- Weakness
- Chest pain radiating to your neck, shoulders, or back
- Trouble breathing or taking deep breaths
- Rapid breathing
- Discomfort that's relieved by sitting or leaning forward
- Fainting, dizziness, and loss of consciousness

COR PULMONEA can be defined as an alteration in the structure (e.g., hypertrophy or dilation) and function of the right ventricular (RV) of the heart caused by a primary disorder of the respiratory system resulting in pulmonary hypertension.
MAJOR CAUSES: 1. Right side heart failure 2. Long-term high blood pressure in the arteries of the lung and 3. The right ventricle of the heart is defective.
Signs/Symptoms: Trouble breathing during exercise, fatigue, lethargy, passing out during exertion (physical or mental effort), chest pain during physical activity. Excess fluid that leads to swelling in the body and lower extremities, swelling in various parts of the body.

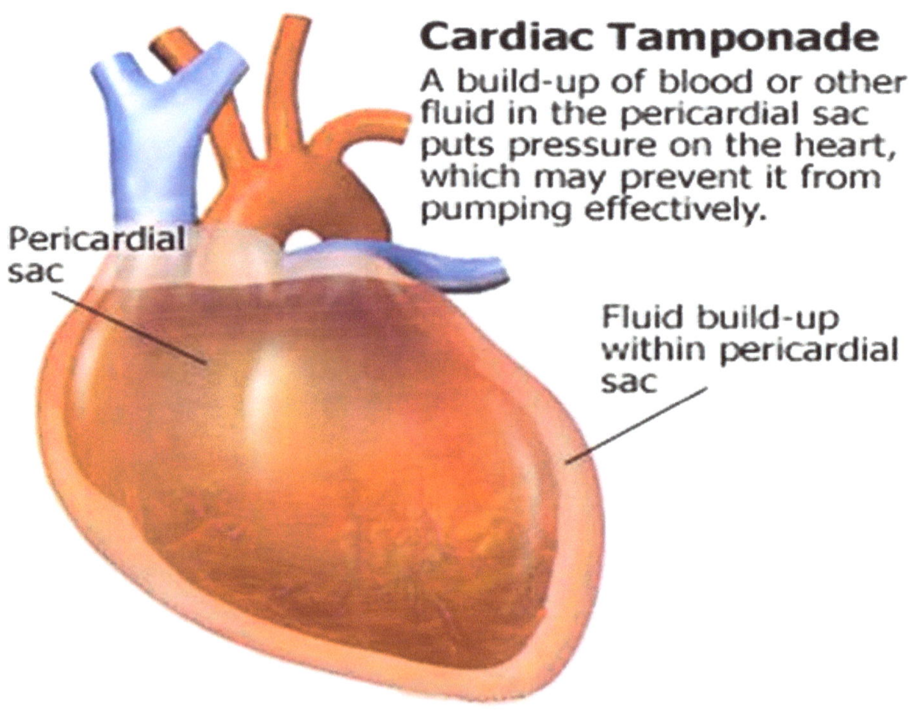

THROMBOSIS:

The formation of a clotted mass of blood within the cardiovascular system.

The clotted mass is thrombus.

[TABLE 4: COLUMN A]

THROMBUS

Involves wall of blood vessels, formed elements of blood and blood clotting system

Composed of platelets and fibrin

May be life threatening

[TABLE 4: COLUMN B]

BLOOD CLOT

Involves only blood clotting system

Composed of fibrin only

Mostly lifesaving

Cause of thrombosis:

Stroke

Myocardial infarction

Pulmonary embolism

Deep vein thrombosis

TENSION PNEUMOTHORAX is a life-threatening condition caused by the continuous entrance and entrapment of air into the pleural space, thereby compressing the lungs, heart, blood vessels, and other structures in the chest.

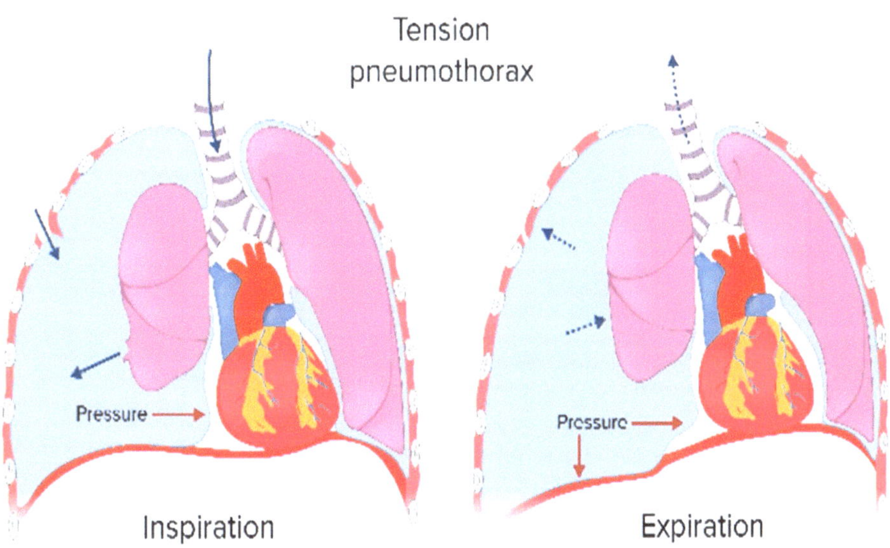

TRAUMA

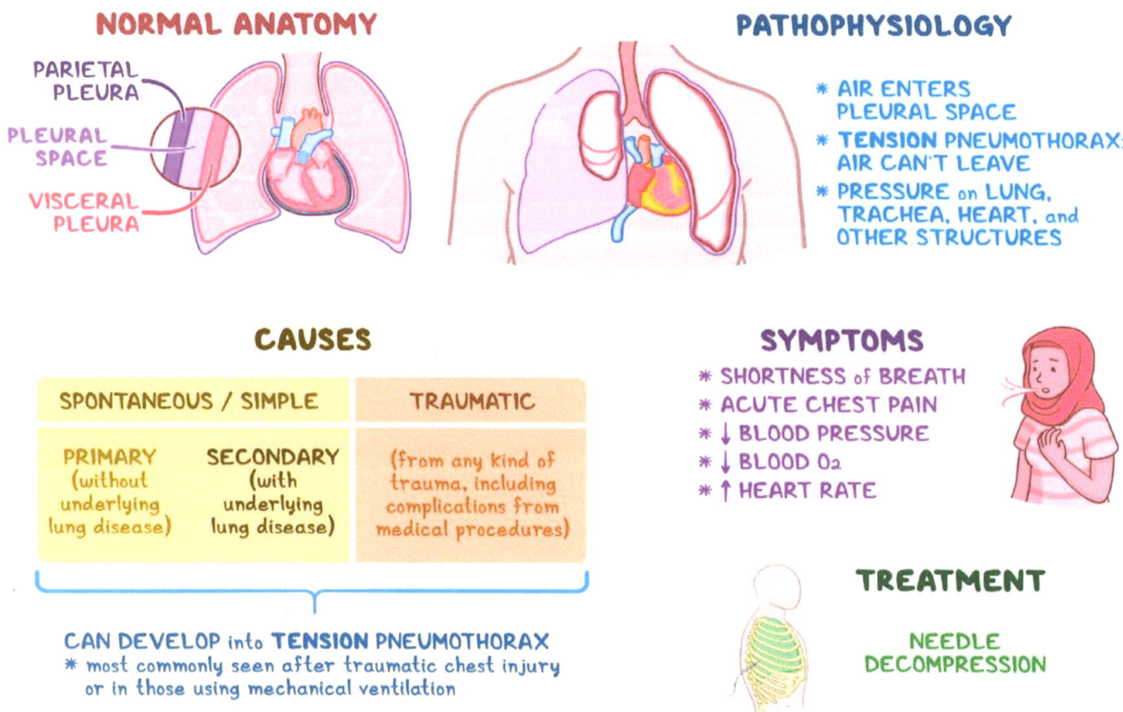

There are three types of traumas: **acute, chronic, or complex**.

Acute trauma is a single event that causes distress or puts you in danger. Acute trauma can include a car accident or a natural disaster.

Chronic trauma is repeated exposure to a dangerous or stressful event, such as bullying or domestic violence.

Complex trauma is repeated exposure to events that cause severe distress or fear such as sexual abuse, torture, or chronic abandonment.

- Migraines
- Nerve damage
- Pain syndromes
- Poor posture
- Surgery
- Trauma
- Toothaches
- Wound cleansing and debridement
- It is important to note that not all analgesics are appropriate for all these conditions.

JACKS NCLEX REVIEW

PHARMACOLOGY REVIEW

PART 2

PHARMACOLOGY STRATEGIES

Anti-Analgesic: Analgesics are medicines that are used to relieve pain. They are also known as painkillers or pain relievers. Technically, the term analgesia refers to a medication that provides relief from pain without putting you to sleep or making you lose consciousness.
Analgesic Medications: Ibuprofen (Advil), Celecoxib (Celebrex), Ketorolac (Sprix (nasal spray)), Naproxen (Aleve), and Indomethacin (Indocin)
What are analgesics used for? Analgesics may be taken to relieve pain that arises from a wide range of conditions, such as:

- Appendicitis; cancer
- Congenital conditions such as curvature of the spine
- Headaches; infection
- Improper lifting techniques
- Menstruation
- Migraines
- Nerve damage
- Pain syndromes
- Poor posture
- Surgery
- Trauma
- Toothaches
- Wound cleansing and debridement
- It is important to note that not all analgesics are appropriate for all these conditions.

Anti-Biotics
Anti-Biotics include medication classifications of aminoglycosides, cephalosporins, macrolides, Lincosamides, penicillin, sulfonamides, tetracyclines, antimycobacterial, and others

Aminoglycosides	Penicillin	Cephalosporins
Amikacin	Amoxicillin	Cefaclor
Gentamicin	Ampicillin	Cefadroxil
Neomycin	Penicillin G	Cefdinir
Streptomycin	Penicillin V	Cefotetan
Tobramycin	Piperacillin	Cefoxitin Ceftriaxone cephalexin

Penicillinase-	Sulfonamides	Fluoroquinolones
➢ Resistant Penicillin's	➢ Sulfamethoxazole	
➢ Dicloxacillin ➢ Nafcillin	➢ Sulfadiazine ➢ Sulfisoxazole	➢ **Fluoroquinolones** ➢ Ofloxacin
➢ oxacillin	➢ Trimethoprim	➢ Ciprofloxacin ➢ Gemifloxacin ➢ Levofloxacin ➢ Moxifloxacin ➢ Norfloxacin

Tetracyclines	**Antimycobacterial**	**Macrolides**	**Monobactam**
Demeclocycline Doxycycline Minocycline Tetracycline	Antituberculosis Leprostatics: clofazimine thalidomide	Azithromycin Clarithromycin erythromycin	aztreonam

Lincosamides	**Antiviral Med.**	**Antifungal Med.**
Clindamycin lincomycin	Acyclovir Foscarnet ganciclovir Valacyclovir	Amphotericin B Fluconazole Itraconazole Ketoconazole Voriconazole

Side Effects of Antibiotics

- Indigestion
- Nausea
- Vomiting
- Bloating
- Diarrhea
- Feeling of fullness
- Stomach pain or cramping
- Loss of appetite

Adverse Effects of Antibiotic

- Ototoxicity, hepatoxicity, nephrotoxicity
- Confusion, disorientation
- Renal toxicity, GI problem
- Palpitations, blood pressure changes
- Hypersensitivity
- Headache, dizziness, lethargy, paresthesia
- Pseudomembranous colitis (cephalosporins, lincosamides)
- Fever, rash, photosensitivity

Adverse Effects of Antibiotic

- Sulfonamides – Bone marrow depression, dermatological effects, including hypersensitivity and photosensitivity, vertigo, ataxia depression, seizure
- Tetracycline - Teeth coloration (staining), dermatological reaction, rash, and photosensitivity

Nursing Considerations for Antibiotics

Aminoglycosides

- Check eight cranial nerve function (hearing)
- Check renal function: BUN and creatinine
- Usually prescribed for seven to ten days
- Encourage fluids
- Small, frequent meals

Nursing considerations for cephalosporins

- Take with food
- Administer liquid form to children; do not crush tablets
- Have vitamin K available for hypoprothrombinemia
- Avoid alcohol while taking medication and for three days after finishing a course of medication
- Cross allergy to penicillin.
- Monitor renal and hepatic function
- Monitor for thrombophlebitis

Nursing considerations of Ciprofloxacin (Cipro), Levofloxacin (Levaquin), and Norfloxacin (Noroxin) => Fluoroquinolones

- Culture and sensitivity before starting therapy
- Take one hour before or two hours after meals with a glass of water
- Encourage fluids
- If needed administer antacids two hours after medication
- Take the full course of therapy

Nursing considerations of Vancomycin (Vancocin) => Glycopeptides

- Monitor renal function and hearing
- Poor absorption orally
- Administer IV: peak five minutes, duration twelve to twenty-four hours
- Avoid extravasation during therapy => necrosis possible
- Give antihistamine if "red man syndrome": decreased blood pressure, flushing of face and neck
- Contact clinician if signs of superinfection: sore throat, fever, fatigue

Nursing considerations of Erythromycin and Azithromycin => Macrolide

- Take oral medication one hour before or two to three hours after meals with a full glass of water.
- Take around the clock to maximize effectiveness.
- Take the full course of therapy.

Nursing considerations of Clindamycin => Lincosamides

- Administer oral med with a full glass of water => prevent ulcers

- Monitor for persistent vomiting, diarrhea, fever, or abdominal pain and cramping, superinfections

Nursing considerations of penicillin

- Culture and sensitivity before treatment
- Monitor serum electrolytes and cardiac status if given IV.
- Monitor and rotate injection sites, monitor for twenty minutes after IM.
- Good mouth care
- One to two hour ac or two to three hour pc => reduce gastric acid destruction
- Yogurt or buttermilk if diarrhea develops => loose, foul-smelling stool
- Instruct patient to take missed drugs as soon as possible; do not double dose.
- Check cross-sensitivity with cephalosporins.
- There are several common side effects associated with penicillin, including nausea, vomiting, gastrointestinal distress, and diarrhea. Moreover, the tongue may become black and hairy as a result of the medication.
- Adverse Effects: Patients should be monitored for C-diff, candidiasis, and hyperkalemia. Other signs of hypersensitivity may include rash (maculopapular to exfoliative dermatitis), urticaria, laryngeal edema, and anaphylaxis.

Nursing considerations of tetracyclines

- Take one hour before or two to three hours after meals.
- GI upset => with food except for milk or food high in calcium
- Do not take antacids, milk, or iron preparations.
- Note expiration date => highly nephrotoxic => I & O
- Protect from sunlight
- Monitor renal function
- Topical applications may stain clothing.
- Use the contraceptive method in addition to oral contraceptives.

Nursing considerations of Sulfisoxazole (Gantrisin) => sulfonamides

- Monitor I and O, force fluids
- Maintain alkaline urine
- Bicarbonate may be indicated to elevate the ph.
- Avoid vitamin C, which acidifies the urine.

Nursing considerations of Sulfasalazine (Azulfidine) => sulfonamides

- Advise clients to avoid exposure to sunlight.
- Maintain fluid intake at 3000 mL/day to avoid crystal formation.

Nursing considerations of Trimethoprim/Sulfamethoxazole (Bactrim, Septra) => sulfonamides

- Obtain C & S before first dose.
- IV solution must be given slowly over sixty to ninety minutes.
- Never administer IM.
- Encourage fluids to 3000/day.

Antibiotics

- Nursing considerations of Doxycycline (Vibramycin) => Tetracyclines
- Check the patient's tongue for Monilia infection.

Antibiotics

Nursing considerations Ciprofloxacin (Cipro) => Fluoroquinolones

- Contraindicated in children < eighteen years old
- Two hours pc or two hours before an antacid or iron preparations
- Avoid caffeine
- Encourage fluids

Anticonvulsants

- CARBAMAZEPINE (Carbatrol, Epitol, Equctro, tegretol, Tegretol XR)
- DIVALPROEX SODIUM (Depakote, Depakote ER)
- GABAPENTIN (Gabarone, Neurontin)
- LAMOTRIGINE (Lamictal)
- PHENOBARBITAL (Luminal)
- PHENYTOIN (Dilantin)
- TOPIRAMATE (Topamax, Topiragen)

CARBAMAZEPINE (Carbatrol, Epitol, Equetro, Tegretol, Tegretol XR)

Side Effects

- Myelosuppression
- Dizziness, drowsiness
- Ataxia
- Diplopia, rash
- Photosensitivity

Anticonvulsants (continued)

CARBAMAZEPINE Side Effects

- Depression
- Nausea
- Vomiting
- Dyspepsia
- Aplastic anemia
- Stevens-Johnson syndrome
- Suicide attempts in bipolar patients

CARBAMAZEPINE Nursing Considerations

- Management of seizures, trigeminal neuralgia, diabetic neuropathy
- Avoid driving and other activities requiring alertness the first three days.
- Monitor blood levels and CBC regularly, especially during the first two months; periodic eye exams

- Take with food or milk to decrease GI upset; tablets (nonextended-release) may be crushed, extended-release capsules may be opened and mixed with juice or soft food (no grapefruit products)
- Urine may turn pink to brown.
- Avoid abrupt withdrawal; discontinue gradually.
- Avoid the use of alcohol and CNS depressants.
- Inform the physician before taking any new medication or herbal medication.
- Rx; Preg Cat D

DIVALPROEX SODIUM (Depakote, Depakote ER) treats:

- Mania associated with bipolar disorder
- Bipolar depression
- Bipolar I disorder with most recent episode mixed
- Bipolar disorder in remission
- Migraine prevention
- A type of seizure disorder called tonic-clonic epilepsy
- Seizures with irregular muscle contractions

ANTICONVULSANTS, DIVALPROEX SODIUM

Side Effects

- Petit mal seizures
- Epilepsy
- Convulsive seizures
- Nausea, vomiting, stomach pain, diarrhea, constipation.
- Headache, back pain
- Dizziness, drowsiness, weakness, tremors
- Memory problems, mood changes, trouble sleeping
- Bruising or bleeding
- Runny nose, sore throat, cough, wheezing, trouble breathing

ANTICONVULSANTS: Side Effects

- Fever, flu symptoms
- Problems with walking or coordination
- Swelling in your hands or feet
- Blurred vision, double vision, unusual eye movements
- Ringing in your ears
- Rach, hair loss; or
- Changes in weight or appetite

Anti-inflammatory Medication – Nonsteroidal Anti-Inflammatories (NSAIDs)

Nonsteroidal anti-inflammatory medications are one of the most used types of medications for musculoskeletal conditions. NSAIDs can be effective for a wide variety of orthopedic conditions from arthritis to tendinitis, or other inflammatory conditions.

The most prescribed or recommended NSAID medications are:

- Bayer, Ecotrin, Bufferin (aspirin)
- Motrin, Advil (ibuprofen)
- Aleve, (Aleve [OTC], Anaprox Naprosyn (naproxen)
- Mobic (Meloxicam)
- Celebrex (celecoxib)
- Methotrexate (Trexall)

Side effects of Naproxen

- GI bleeding
- Blood dyscrasias
- Hives
- Rash
- Asthma

NURSE CONSIDERATION OF NAPROXEN

Management of mild to moderate pain; treatment of rheumatoid, juvenile, and gouty arthritis, osteoarthritis, primary dysmenorrhea

Patients with asthma, ASA hypersensitivity, or nasal polyps have an increased risk of hypersensitivity

- Contact clinician if blurred vision, ringing, or roaring in ears, which may indicate toxicity.
- Contact clinician if black stools, flulike symptoms.
- Contact clinician if changes in urinary pattern, increased weight, edema, increased pain in joints, fever, blood in urine, which may indicate kidney damage.
- Use sunscreen to prevent photosensitivity.
- Avoid the use of ASA, steroids, and alcohol.
- OTC, Rx; Preg Cat C

Anti-inflammatory Medication – Nonsteroidal Anti-Inflammatories (NSAIDs)

- A good place to start is with the R.I.C.E. treatment, which stands for:
- Rest
- Ice
- Compression
- Elevation
- Other treatments that may be helpful include certain foods and supplements, topical treatments, and physical activities.

- An often-neglected method to control inflammation is rest. Getting enough overall rest and sleep and taking it easy on the injured part of your body allows the inflammation to subside and the recovery process to unfold.

Anti-inflammatory medication – nonsteroidal anti-inflammatory drugs

Not only does this mean resting from athletics, but often this means allowing an injured body part to rest from normal activities that may prolong inflammation. If you have a busy life, rest might not be built into your routine, but ignoring the signs of inflammation may prolong the problem.

Side Effects of NSAIDs

- Bleeding risks
- Kidney problem
- Stomach upset/ulcer
- Hypertension/stroke
- NSAID medications have potential side effects, even those that can be obtained over the counter. Some of the side effects are minor, and others are potentially dangerous.

SIDE EFFECTS OF (NSAIDS) NABUMETONE

- Abdominal pain
- Constipation
- Diarrhea
- Flatulence
- Tinnitus
- Edema
- Headache
- Rash
- Gastritis

Nursing Considerations for NSAIDs NABUMETONE

- Used to manage symptoms of osteoarthritis and rheumatoid
- Arthritis
- Take food or milk.
- Contraindicated in patients with hypersensitivity to other NSAIDs
- Alcohol may increase ulcerogenic effects if used concurrently.
- May take two weeks or more to notice improvement.
- Rx; Pregnancy Category C

SIDE EFFECTS OF IBUPROFEN

- Headache
- Nausea, anorexia
- GI bleeding
- Blood dyscrasias

- Hives
- Facial swelling
- Rash
- Side

NURSING CONSIDERATIONS OF IBUPROFEN

- Treatment of rheumatoid arthritis, osteoarthritis, primary dysmenorrhea, gout, dental pain, musculoskeletal disorders, fever, headache, menstrual cramps
- Onset: thirty minutes, peak one to two hours
- Full therapeutic effect may take up to one month.
- Contact clinician if blurred vision, ringing or roaring in ears, which may indicate toxicity.
- Contact clinician if changes in urinary pattern increased weight, edema, increased pain in joints, fever, and blood in urine, which may indicate kidney damage.
- Avoid use with ASA, NSAIDs, and alcohol, which may precipitate.
- GI bleeding
- Take food or milk.
- Possible cross-allergy with aspirin
- OTC, Rx; Preg Cat C

- **Antineoplastics**
- **Methotrexate**
- **Tamoxifen**

Antineoplastic drugs are medications used to treat cancer. Antineoplastic drugs are also called anticancer, chemotherapy, chemo, cytotoxic, or hazardous drugs.

Antineoplastics

SIDE EFFECTS OF METHOTREXATE

- Nausea, vomiting, diarrhea
- Anorexia
- Alopecia
- Ulcerative stomatitis
- Dizziness
- Side

Antineoplastic

NURSE CONSIDERATION OF METHOTREXATE

- Treatment of cancer, mycosis fungoides, psoriasis, rheumatoid arthritis
- PO, IM, IV: onset four to seven days, peak seven to fourteen days, duration twenty-one days

- Avoid crowds and people with known infections.
- Do not take acetylsalicylic acid (ASA) or other NSAIDs, which may cause GI bleeding.
- Monitor for pulmonary toxicity, which may manifest early as a dry, nonproductive cough.
- Rx; Pregnancy Category X

SIDE EFFECTS OF TAMOXIFEN

- Nausea, vomiting
- Hot flashes
- Rash
- Vaginal discharge
- Irregular menses
- Fluid retention
- Depression, mood disturbances

Nursing Considerations of Tamoxifen

- Management of advanced breast cancer not responsive to other therapy in estrogen-receptor-positive patients
- Peak four to seven hours
- To decrease GI upset, take after antacid, after an evening meal, before bedtime, or take antiemetic thirty to sixty minutes ahead.
- Vaginal bleeding, pruritus, and hot flashes are reversible after stopping the medication.
- Contact clinician if decreased visual acuity, which may be irreversible.
- Tumor flares (increase in tumor size and increased bone pain) may occur but will decrease rapidly; may take analgesics for pain.
- Rx; Preg Cat D

Anti-Inflammatory Medications such as **Corticosteroids**

- HYDROCORTISONE (Cortef, Solu-Cortef)
- METHYLPREDNISOLONE (Medrol)
- PREDNISONE (Deltasone, Meticorten, Prednisone Intensol)

SIDE EFFECTS OF HYDROCORTISONE

- Depression
- Flushing, sweating
- Hypertension
- Nausea, diarrhea
- Hyperglycemia
- Psychic derangements

Nursing Considerations for HYDROCORTISONE

- Treatment of severe inflammation, septic shock, adrenal insufficiency, ulcerative colitis, collagen disorders
- Medication masks signs of infection, so check for elevated temperature, WBC count
- PO: take with food, milk, antacids

- IM: give deep into gluteal UOQ, avoid deltoid, rotate sites, and avoid subQ administration because it may damage tissue
- Monitor blood sugar in diabetes carefully.
- Rectal: for colitis, retain medication for twenty minutes, onset three to five days
- Wear medical information tag.
- Do not mix with other medicines.
- Rx; Preg Category C

SIDE EFFECTS FOR METHYLPREDNISOLONE

- Peptic ulcer/possible perforation
- Hypertension and circulatory problems
- Poor wound healing
- Hyperglycemia
- Psychic derangements

Anti-Inflammatory Medications such as CORTICOSTEROIDS

Nursing Considerations

- Treatment of severe inflammation, shock, adrenal insufficiency, management of acute spinal cord injury, collagen disorders
- PO: take with food, milk, antacids
- PO: peak one to two hours, duration 1.5 days
- IM: give deep into gluteal UOQ, avoid deltoid, rotate sites, avoid subQ administration because it may damage tissue
- IM: peak four to eight days, duration one to four weeks

Nursing Consideration METHYLPREDNISOLONE

- Eat food high in protein, calcium, and vitamin D; avoid sodium.
- Contact clinician if anorexia, difficulty breathing, weakness, dizziness.
- Symptoms may appear during periods of stress or trauma.
- Contact clinician if black/tarry stools, slow wound healing, blurred vision, bruising/bleeding, weight gain, emotional changes
- Wear medical information tag.
- Monitor patient weight, blood sugar
- Rx; Pregnancy Category C

SIDE EFFECTS OF PREDNISONE

- Depression
- Hypertension, circulatory problems
- Nausea, diarrhea
- Abdominal distention

Nursing Considerations for PREDNISONE

- Treatment of severe inflammation, immunosuppression, neoplasms
- PO: take with food, milk, antacids

- PO: peak one to two hours, duration three to thirty-six hours
- IM: give deep into gluteal UOQ, avoid deltoid, rotate sites, and avoid subcutaneous administration because it may damage the tissue.
- IM: peak one hour, duration four weeks
- Eat food high in protein, calcium, and vitamin D; avoid sodium.
- Contact clinician if anorexia, difficulty breathing, weakness, or dizziness; symptoms may appear during periods of stress or trauma.
- Contact clinician if black/tarry stools, slow wound healing, blurred vision, bruising/bleeding, weight gain, emotional changes.
- Wear medical information tag.
- Rx; Pregnant Category C

CARDIOVASCULAR DISORDER / MEDICATIONS:

This is also called heart disease.
Treatments vary widely and can include lifestyle changes, medications, surgery, stents, pacemakers, and ablation.

MEDICAL SURGICAL

Topics:

- Cardiovascular Disorders
- Angina
- Myocardial Infarction
- Heart Failure
- Endocarditis
- Valve Replacement
- Hypertension
- Hypertension Crisis
- Peripheral Arterial Disease (Pad)
- Abdominal Aortic Aneurysm (AAA)
- Raynaud Disease
- Buerger's Disease

CARDIOVASCULAR DISORDERS

Coronary Artery Disease: this is when lipid fat or CAD sits on the lining of the Heart. It is called hyperlipidemia because of atherosclerosis.

Causes:

- Not eating healthy food
- Hypertension
- Diabetes
- Overweight (obesity)
- Physical inactivity
- Smoking tobacco
- Family history of heart disease

Coronary Artery Disease (CAD): this is when lipid fat or CAD sits on the lining of the Heart. It is called hyperlipidemia because of atherosclerosis.

Causes:

- Not eating healthy food
- Hypertension
- Diabetes
- Overweight (obesity)
- Physical inactivity
- Smoking tobacco
- Family history of heart disease

Coronary Artery Disease

Diet:

- Low cholesterol food
- High fiber food

Signs and symptoms:

- Chest pain
- Shortness of breath
- Tachycardia
- Gastrointestinal indigestion or nausea
- Lightheadedness or sweating

Goals for Coronary Artery Disease patient:

The goal is to give the patient anti-lipid meds that will help and break the lipid. However, the drugs are called "statins" medication such as:

- Atorvastatin (Lipitor)
- Fluvastatin (Lescol)
- Lovastin (Mevacor)
- Pravastatin (Pravachol)
- Simvastatin (zocor)

Side effects and adverse effects of statin meds

Side effects	**Adverse effects**
Headache	Statin causes leg cramps
Dizziness	Statin destroys your eyes
Feeling sick	Must be given in the evening

- Feeling unusually tired or physically weak, low blood platelet count
- Cannot be taken for more than 2-3 months
- Digestive system problems: constipation, diarrhea, indigestion, or farting
- It destroys your liver, increase the risk for myoditics
- Muscle pain
- Myalgias
- Sleep problems   rhbdomyolysis

Patient Teaching:

Teach patient to undergo liver enzymes test

Inform patient to take HmG-CoA reductase inhibitors- statin class of drugs that is lipid-lowering meds that reduce illness and mortality in those who are at high risk of cardiovascular disease.

ANGINA

This simple means Chest Pain caused by reduced blood flow to the heart and resulting from myocardial ischemia caused by inadequate myocardial blood and oxygen supply.

Types of ANGINAS

1. Stable Angina (chest pain) because of some forms of activities, you are doing e.g. cooking, dancing, you can have chest pain in that process. Chest pain is also called exertion angina.

Nursing Intervention:

- Nurse will administer the patient:
- Rest, oxygen, and nitroglycerin.
- **Note**: nitroglycerin is vasodilator: it can treat and prevent chest pain (angina) in its oral form. When used rectally, it can treat pain caused by tears in the skin around the opening for bowel movements (anal fissures).
- Given under the tongue (sublingual).
- Check the patient's blood pressure and heart rate.
- Check the patient's heart rate.
- Different between Angina and MI

ANGINA (chest pain) /MYOCARDIA INFARCTION

ANGINA(Chest Pain) Can develop slowly or quickly.Radiate to the shoulders, arms, jaw, neck, and back.Occurs without cause, usually early in the morning Crushing substernal pain-The chest pain radiate to the left arm back, and jaw Mild or moderate pain, substernal, crushing, squeezing painLasts less than 5 minutes, however, can last up to 15-20 minutes Treat with nitroglycerin or rest and oxygen.	MYOCARDIA INFARCTION Happens without a cause, essentially early in the morning crushing substernal pain radiate to the jaw, back, and left armLasts 30 minutes or longerUnrelieved by rest or nitroglycerin, Only relieved by opioid.

2. Unstable chest pain: patient have the chest pain while on rest, watching TV. This is a bad sign.

Nursing Intervention

Treat with rest, oxygen, give 1 nitroglycerin (under the tongue) wait for 5 mins. Then give second nitroglycerin check vital signs wait for 5 mins. Then the third nitroglycerin, check vital sign and if it does not resolve or go away and the chest pain continued call 911. The reason is because the patient might be developing MI which also called Heart attack.

3. Variant Angina- this is always bad it is also called Prinzmetal's or vasospastic angina. It is also a result from coronary artery disease. May occur at rest usually at night. Attach may be associated with ST segment elevation noted on the electrocardiogram.

Myocardial Infarction:

Anytime patient have MI, know that it is medical emergency. MI occurs when myocardial tissue is unexpectedly dies and have a being severely deprived of oxygen. Location of MI obstruction of the left anterior descending artery results in anterior or septal MI or both

Risks Factors

- Atherosclerosis
- Coronary artery disease elevated cholesterol levels
- Smoking
- Hypertension
- Obesity
- Physical inactivity
- Impaired glucose tolerance
- stress

Diagnostic studies/Labs:

- Troponin- This blood test for MI
- Creatine kinase Level
- CK-MB Isoenzyme
- Myoglobin
- IDH Level
- White Blood Count
- electro diagram

Sign and Symptoms of MI

- Pain
- Nausea and vomiting
- Diaphoresis
- Dyspnea
- Dysrhythmias
- Feeling of fear and anxiety
- Pallor, cyanosis. And coolness of extremities

Complication of MI

- Dysrhythmias
- Heart Failure
- Pulmonary edema
- Cardiogenic shock

- Thrombophlebitis
- Pericarditis
- Mitral valve insufficiency
- Postinfarction Angina
- Ventricular rupture

Nursing Intervention, acute stage

- Obtain a detail history of the chest discomfort.
- Assess vital signs
- Assess cardiovascular status and maintain cardiac monitor (e.k.g.)
- Place the patient in semi-fowler's position to enhance comfort and tissue oxygenation
- Administer oxygen at 2 to 4 l/min by nasal cannula as prescribed
- Establish an IV access route.
- For the RN- Give oxygen first before giving other meds
- For the Physician order- give OMNA:

O= Oxygen

M= Morphine

N= Nitroglycerin

A= Aspirin

Obtain 12 lead electrocardiogram.

Heart Failure this is a pumping problem that means the heart cannot pump enough oxygen-rich blood to meet the body's needs. Also, without enough blood flow, the organs may not function properly which will lead to serious problem.

Types of Heart Failure

Left-side Heart Failure – all the problems will be **respiratory** related.

Right-side Heart Failure- all the problems will be **fluid and blood** in the body.

LEFT SIDE HEART FAILURE (S/S)

- Awakening at night with shortness of breath
- Coughing Wheezing

- Difficult concentrating
- dizziness
- Fatigue
- Tachycardia
- dyspnea
- crackle in the lungs

RIGHT SIDE HEART FAILURE (S/S)

- Shortness of breath during exercise or lying flat
- Difficult concentrating,
- Fatigue, anorexia and nausea
- Hypertension (Increase BP)
- nocturnal diuresis
- Fluid retention causing swelling
- Weight gain
- Bradycardia,
- Decrease BP (from pump Failure

Nursing Intervention/Management of heart failure.

- Place the patient in high flower's position, with the legs in a dependent position, to reduce pulmonary congestion and relieve swelling (edema).
- Administer oxygen in high concentrations by mask or cannula as per MD orders to improve gas exchange and pulmonary function.
- Get patient ready for intubation and ventilator support if required.
- Monitor lung sounds for crackles and decreased breath sounds.
- suction fluids ad needed to maintain a patent airway
- assess patient for level of consciousness
- monitor patient's vital signs closely
- Monitor intake and output (I&O)

Treatment of Heart Failure

- Digoxin treats Heart Failure and Heart rhythm problems.
- Check heart rate before administering med.
- Heart Rate / pulse must be 60 bpm if less please HOLD digoxin.
- Too much digoxin – causes toxicity / overdose
- Give Lasix – to remove excess fluid in the body.

Sign/Symptoms of digoxin toxicity or overdose.

- GI problems- vomiting, diarrhea, nausea
- Eye problem
- Anytime these happened you must stop the drug and call the Doctor.
- Antidote/reversal medication for digoxin is called Digibind.
- If you give too much digoxin- patient potassium will go low
- If you give too little digoxin- the patient potassium will go high

Nursing Intervention

Monitor patients' potassium level because Lasix can cause the patient to void too much urine and waste the potassium in the body.

- Weigh patient daily
- Limit fluid
- Watch patient intake of salt.
- Watch patient diet.
- Encourage patient to walk around.
- Watch patient activity level to avoid shortness of breath.
- Patient may feel dizzy.
- Avoid stress.
- Exercise to keep fit e.g., isometric.

Lab test/ diagnostic studies

BNP – best for Heart Failure. Normal level of BNP is 100 pg/mL. if BNP is great than 100 pg/mL that is an indication of **heart failure**.

Valve Replacement

This is called a procedure where a defective heart valve is removed and replaced with a new one. It is a major surgical procedure and is usually recommended when other less invasive treatments such as medication and lifestyle changes are not effective. Valve replacement is usually performed under general anesthesia and involves an open-heart surgery. The new valve is then implanted, and sutures are used to secure it in place. After the procedure, the patient will be kept in the hospital for observation.

Types of valve replacement include open heart surgery, minimally invasive valve surgery, and transcatheter valve replacement. Valve replacement is a serious procedure and should only be performed by an experienced cardiac surgeon. Open heart surgery involves making a large incision in the chest to access the heart and valves. Minimally invasive valve surgery requires only a small incision in the chest. Transcatheter valve replacement involves inserting a catheter through a blood vessel to access the heart and valves.

Peripheral Arterial Disease (Pad)

Peripheral Arterial Disease (Pad) is a condition that affects the arteries in the legs and other parts of the body.

- It can cause pain, fatigue, and numbness in the legs and feet.
- If left untreated, it can lead to more serious health problems.
- Treatment for Pad usually involves lifestyle changes, such as quitting smoking, exercising regularly, and maintaining a healthy blood pressure. In some cases, medication or medical procedures may be necessary.
- Surgery may be needed to remove part or all the prostate glands.
- Radiation therapy may also be used to treat severe cases of Pad.
- Surgery and radiation therapy can have serious side effects, so it is important for patients to discuss them with their healthcare provider.
- Treatment for Pad should be tailored to the individual's needs and preferences.
- Treatment may include lifestyle modifications, such as quitting smoking or reducing stress.
- Additionally, physical therapy may help to improve urination and pelvic floor muscle health.
- Regular check-ups are also important to monitor the progress of treatment.

Abdominal Aortic Aneurysm (AAA)

Abdominal aortic aneurysm is an enlargement of the aorta, the main artery in the human body. It is caused by weakening of the artery walls and can lead to rupture or blockage. Treatment usually involves surgical repair. Aortic aneurysms are serious and can be life-threatening if not treated quickly. Regular check-ups and screenings can help detect aneurysms before they become too large and serious.

Who are at risk. The risk of an aortic aneurysm increases with age and family history. People with high blood pressure, high cholesterol, and smoking habits are also more likely to develop an aortic aneurysm. Especially African Americans who do not take their blood pressure medications.

It is important for the patient to take their BP medications for the rest of their lives as long as possible.

Regular exercise and a healthy diet can also reduce the risk of aortic aneurysms. People with a family history of aortic aneurysms should get regular medical check-ups to monitor their health.

Signs and symptoms of Abdominal aortic aneurysm Abdominal aortic aneurysms can cause sudden, severe, and constant pain; a pulsating sensation in the abdomen; and difficulty breathing. Syncope, dyspnea, hoarseness, and difficulty swallowing are all symptoms of aneurysm pressure.

Raynaud Disease

This is a vasospasm or disorder where the blood is not flowing through the arteries in your hands, face, cheek bones and ears. This disease is genetic. There is a high incidence of this disease among white girls who smoke (also known as the red, white and blue disease). The patient's hands, ears, or check will be red, then white, and then blue, which is called cyanotic, requiring an amputation.

- Treatment usually involves vasodilators, such as nitroglycerin or papaverine, to help relax the muscles in the arteries. Surgery may be necessary in some cases.
- Procardia- Calcium channel blocker- this is a vasodilator medication.
- Teaching: - is mostly for prevention purposes
- Make sure the patient wears gloves, mittens, covers up, does not smoke, and takes blood pressure medications.
- Always keep your fingers and hands warm.

Buerger's Disease

Buerger's disease this disease is also known as (thromboangitis Obliterans) affects blood vessels in the body, most commonly in the arms and legs. It is caused by smoking and can lead to permanent tissue damage, pain, gangrene and amputation.

Treatment usually involves quitting smoking, wearing compression stockings, and medication to reduce swelling and inflammation. Surgery may also be necessary in some cases. Early diagnosis and treatment are essential for reducing permanent damage.

Hypertension

Hypertension

There are two types of hypertensions: primary hypertension and secondary hypertension. Primary hypertension is the most common and is caused by genetics, lifestyle, and age. Secondary hypertension is caused by an underlying medical condition, such as kidney disease or sleep apnea.

Treatment for both types involve lifestyle changes such as exercise and diet, as well as medications. Regular blood pressure monitoring is also recommended to keep track of blood pressure levels. Other lifestyle changes include quitting smoking and reducing alcohol intake. Some people may also benefit from stress management techniques. Regular visits to the doctor are important for on-going monitoring and advice.

Primary hypertension: another name is Essential.

- Genetic
- Black American
- Smokers
- Obesity
- Immobility
- Lack of exercise
- Diabetes
- Stress and excessive alcohol
- Hyperlipidemia
- Increase intake of salt or caffeine
- Sentinel lifestyle

The patient with secondary hypertension has a disorder that leads to hypertension. For example, when a patient has a kidney disorder, this kidney disorder may contribute to hypertension. Also, a patient who is pregnant and has preeclampsia that leads to gestational hypertension.

Classification of hypertension

Pre-hypertension

Stage 1

Stage 2

Nursing intervention in prehypertension: education on lifestyle changes. This includes reducing salt intake, increasing physical activity, and quitting smoking. Additionally, regular blood pressure checks are advised.

Nursing intervention stage 1: education on lifestyle changes. Education on lifestyle changes is important because it can help individuals make the necessary lifestyle changes to reduce blood pressure. Additionally, regular blood pressure checks are important to ensure that any changes are working and that further interventions are necessary. Also, at this stage the physician can place the patient on Beta blocker medication e.g. Procardia (Calcium Channel Blocker).

Nursing intervention stage 2 involves administering Beta blocker medication and monitoring the patient's blood pressure. The nurse should also monitor the patient's heart rate and any side effects that the medication may cause. Finally, the nurse should provide education and support to the patient on lifestyle changes. The physician can also order angiotensin converting enzyme inhibitor (ACE)- relaxes the veins and arteries to lower blood pressure. This medication's last name ends in ...Pril.

Adverse Effect of ACE Inhibitors - ACE inhibitors can cause a dry cough, dizziness, and kidney problems. It is important to monitor the patient's kidney function while taking this medication. ACE inhibitors work by blocking an enzyme that increases blood pressure. This blockage can cause a decrease in the amount of fluid in the blood, leading to dehydration and kidney problems. In addition, ACE inhibitors can cause a dry cough and dizziness.

Nursing Intervention/Teaching:

Nursing intervention/teaching should include patient education on how to recognize signs of dehydration, such as dry mouth, fatigue, and increased thirst, and when to seek medical attention. Nurses should also inform patients that ACE inhibitors can cause a dry cough and dizziness and advise them to take regular breaks throughout the day to reduce the risk of dizziness.

Hypertension Crisis

Hypertension crisis occurs when blood pressure rises to 200/100. This is a medical emergency. A crisis in hypertension is usually caused by a sudden increase in blood pressure, which can cause damage to the heart, kidneys, and brain. It is important to seek medical attention immediately to prevent serious health complications.

Treatment for hypertension crisis usually involves medication, lifestyle changes, and stress management. In some cases, hospitalization may be necessary. Medication can help to lower blood pressure, while lifestyle changes such as reducing sodium intake and increasing physical activity can help to manage stress. In severe cases, hospitalization may be necessary to monitor blood pressure and provide further treatment if necessary.

It is important to see this patient first. Also, this patient will no longer receives PO medications. They will only get IV medications.

Medication for patients with hypertensive crisis includes:

- Nitroprusside - IV BP Med.
- Phentolamine or Regitine BP Med.

Side Effects of Nitroprusside include dizziness, confusion, headache, blurred vision, and nausea. It can also cause low blood pressure, bradycardia, and hypotension. It can also cause allergic reactions such as hives, difficulty breathing, swelling of the face, lips, tongue, and throat.

Nursing Intervention/Teaching

Do not use nitroprusside if the patient has hereditary vision loss. To avoid Leber's' disease. Nitroprusside can cause damage to the retina, which can lead to hereditary vision loss. Leber's disease is a rare genetic disorder that can lead to vision loss.

Continuous monitoring of blood pressure, telemetry and urine output is essential.

Angiotensin Converting Enzyme Inhibitors: (ACE) inhibitors prevent peripheral vasoconstriction by blocking the conversion of angiotensin II (AII).
ACE Inhibitor is used to treat hypertension and heart failure.
AVOID using ACE with potassium supplements and potassium-retaining (sparing) diuretics.

What are the most common ACE inhibitors Medications?

- Benazepril (Lotensin, LotensinHct)
- Captopril (Capoten)
- Enalapril (Vasotec)
- Eosinopril (Monopril)
- Lisinopril (Prinivil, Zestril)
- Moexopril (Univasc)
- Perindopril (Aceon)
- Quinapril (Accupril)

What are ACE inhibitors used to treat? ACE inhibitors are used to prevent, treat, or improve symptoms in conditions such as:

- High blood pressure (hypertension)
- Coronary artery disease
- Heart failure
- Diabetes
- Certain chronic kidney diseases
- Heart attacks
- A disease that involves hardening of the skin and connective tissues (scleroderma)

- Migraines

Side effects of ACE inhibitors may include:

- Dry cough
- Increased potassium levels in the blood (hyperkalemia)
- Fatigue
- Dizziness from blood pressure going too low
- Headaches
- Loss of taste

Nursing Intervention ACE INHIBITORS

Monitor the client's BP; if less than 90/60 mm Hg, hold and question the order.
Instruct the client to contact the doctor if there is a persistent dry cough.
Teach the client about orthostatic hypotension.
Instruct the client to stop the medication suddenly (abruptly).
Nurse teachings
Monitor potassium levels; it can cause a rise in potassium levels.

PRACTICE QUESTION

The health care provider ordered Lisinopril an angiotensin-converting enzyme (ACE) inhibitor for a client diagnosed with CHF. Which instruction should the nurse provide?
"Eat a banana or drink orange juice at least twice a day."
"Notify the HCP if you develop bruising or petechiae." Correct!
"Expect to have a persistent dry cough early in the morning on arising."
"Your symptoms of congestive heart failure should improve rapidly."

Angiotensin II receptor blockers (ARBS)

Angiotensin II is a type of peptide/protein hormone that narrows the blood vessels to control blood pressure and fluid balance in the body. Hence, these are being used to treat high blood pressure and heart failure.
This angiotensin-II has an effect to increase the blood pressure, body fluid, and sodium content. Hence, -sartans are being used to treat high blood pressure and heart failure.
MEDS: Losartan, Valsartan

Angiotensin II Receptors Blockers (ARBS)

Nursing Intervention

Monitor the client's BP; if less 90/60 mm Hg, hold and question the order.
Notify HCP when holding because it is cardio-protective and the drug may be given for reasons other than BP. HCP will provide a set of parameters for holding.

Teach the client about orthostatic hypotension.
Instruct the client to discontinue medications abruptly.

ANTIDYSRHTHMIC MEDICATIONS
Class IA- quinidine (Quindex), procainamide
Class IB- lidocaine, Phenytoin (Dilantin)
Class IC- flecainide (Tambocor)
Class II- propranolol
Class III- amiodarone
Class IV- diltiazem (Cardizem) verapamil (Calan)
Reduces automaticity, slows conduction of electrical impulses through the heart, and prolongs the refractory period of myocardial cells (suppress dysrhythmias)

ANTIDYSRHYTHMIC MEDICATION Nursing Consideration
Take an apical pulse rate before administering the drug.
Notify the HCP if the rate falls below sixty beats per minute (bpm) for adults.
Teach the client to monitor and record his pulse.
Make sure the client is being closely monitored on telemetry, with frequent BP monitoring; when administering IV, do not leave the client (administer via infusion pump).
Monitor serum drug levels to maintain therapeutic range.

BETA BLOCKER ADRENERGICS
Dobutamine: increases myocardial force and cardiac output through stimulation of - receptors
Dopamine: increase BP and cardiac output through positive inotropic action and increases renal blood flow through its action on - and - receptors
Epinephrine: used for cardiac stimulation in cardiac arrest, used for bronchodilation in asthma or allergic reactions
Acebutolol, Atenolol, Metoprolol, Propranolol, Bisoprolol
Purpose: used to lower blood pressure and heart rate
Possible side effects, interactions, and special instructions: dizziness, fatigue, dry mouth, slow heart rate, weight gain, cold hands and feet. May reduce side effects if taken with food.

PRACTICE QUESTION

The nurse is preparing to hang a dopamine drip for the client who has just been successfully resuscitated. The client is receiving lidocaine 2 mg/min in the existing IV site. Which intervention should the nurse implement when hanging the dopamine drip?
a Initiate another IV line to administer the dopamine drip. Correct!

b Piggyback the dopamine drip in the lidocaine tubing.
c Question the order because dopamine cannot be administered with lidocaine.
d Prepare to help the HCP insert a subclavian line for the dopamine drip.

ANTIPLATELET MEDICATIONS
Adenosine Diphosphate (ADP)
Clopidogrel
Prasugrel
Aspirin

Antiplatelet Purpose: To thin the blood and help prevent and dissolve clots in arteries and stents.
Possible side effects, intersection, and special instructions
I have stomach pain, headache, dizziness, and breathing difficulties.
The side effects are more severe in patients with asthma and allergies.
Take with food.

ANTIPLATELET MEDICATIONS
Aspirin: used to prevent and dissolve clots in the arteries.
Possible side effects, interactions, and special instructions: Stomach upset, headache, and drowsiness. An allergic reaction could cause breathing difficulties and risk of upset stomachs. Other severe side effects include blood in the stool or coughing blood. Take with food to reduce.

Clot Busters (Thrombolytics) Medications:
Activase alteplase, Cathflo Activiuase, Defibrotide defifelio, Retavase, Reteplase, Tenecteplase
Purpose: used to restore blood flow during a heart attack or stroke and to break up blood clots in the legs (deep vein thrombosis)
Possible side effects, interactions, and special instructions: bleeding, abnormal heartbeat, new clotting

ANTICOAGULANT MEDICATIONS.
- COUMADIN (warfarin)
- HAPERIN
- RIVAROXABAN (Xarelto)
- DABIGATRAN (Pradaxa)
- APIXABAN (Eliquis)
- EDOXABAN (Lixiana)
-

ANTICOAGULANT MEDS. (contd.)
- Purpose: to prevent blood clots from forming in the arteries and heart
- Possible side effects, interactions, and special Instructions such as

- bleeding, vomiting or coughing blood, blood in stool, headaches, and dizziness. Do not take aspirin unless directed by the doctor.

CARDIAC GLYCOSIDE MEDICATIONS

- DIGOXIN treats atrial fibrillation and heart failure. The brand names include: (Lanoxicaps, Lanoxin, Digitek) normal level 0.5 – 2 ng/mL.
- Purpose: used to improve your heart's ability to pump blood and helps to slow down an irregular heartbeat
- Possible side effects: side effects are more common if too much is taken and may include nausea, vomiting

Side effects: diarrhea, stomach Pain, loss of appetite, unusual tiredness, slow heartbeat, drowsiness Bradycardia, visual disturbance: diplopia, blurred vision, yellow-green halos, and photophobia Take on an empty stomach; high-fiber foods can decrease their absorption.

INTERVENTION/DIGOXIN MEDICATIONS

- Monitor for toxicity as evidenced by anorexia, nausea, vomiting, visual disturbance, confusion, bradycardia, heart block, tachydysrhythmias.
- Therapeutic level of digoxin ranges is 0.5 to 2 mg/mL

INTERVENTION/DIGOXIN MEDICATION

- An increased risk of toxicity exists in clients with hypercalcemia, hypokalemia, hypomagnesemia, or hypothyroidism.
- Monitor potassium level; if hypokalemia occurs, notify the physician.
- Instruct the client to avoid over-the-counter medications.
- Monitor the client taking a potassium-wasting diuretic or corticosteroids closely for hypokalemia because the hypokalemia can cause digoxin toxicity.
- The older clients are more sensitive to digoxin toxicity.
- Advise the clients to eat food high in potassium, such as fresh and dried fruits, fruit juices, vegetables, and potatoes.

INTERVENTION/DIGOXIN MEDICATION (continued)

- Monitor the apical pulse/heart rate.
- Assess the heart rate before administering. If HR is less than 60 bpm, hold the medication and notify the HCP.
- Teach the client how to measure pulse.
- Teach the client to notify the physician if the pulse rate is less than 60 bpm or greater than 100 bpm.
- Teach the client the signs and symptoms of toxicity.

- The antidote for digoxin is called DIGIBIND. Digibind is used in extreme toxicity. (Digoxin immune fab) contains antigen binding fragments and is used as an antidote to treat a life-threatening overdose of digoxin or digitoxin.

SMOKING CESSATION MEDICATION

- BRUPROPION SR, VARENICLINE
- Purpose: used to make it easier to stop smoking
- Possible side effects/teaching: headaches, problems sleeping, sleepiness, and strange dreams
- Constipation, intestinal gas, nausea, and change in taste
- Depressed mood, thoughts of suicide and attempted suicide
- Teach the client to notify the physician if they have any of these symptoms.

ANTICHOLESTEROL MEDICATIONS

- Atorvastatin (Lipitor)
- Fluvastatin (Lescol)
- Lovastatin (Pravachol)
- Rosuvastatin Calcium (Crestor)
- Simvastatin (Zocor)

Purpose: used to lower your cholesterol level and reduce the risk of heart attacks and strokes
Side effects: muscle pain, liver damage, memory loss nausea, gas, diarrhea, constipation, and rash
Nursing Intervention/Management:

- Teach client to take STATIN meds as prescribed.
- Become physically active.
- Statin can make clients become physically active.
- Do not smoke.
- Control your BP and monitor at home.
- Instruct clients to control their blood sugar.
- Follow up with the physician.
- Reduce body weight and eat a low-fat diet.

CALCIUM CHANNEL BROCKERS MEDICATIONS

- AMLODIPINE (NORVASC, AMVAZ)
- DILTIAZEM
- FELODIPINE
- ISRADIPINE
- NIFEDIPINE
- VERAPOMIL

Purpose: used to decrease cardiac contractility (negative inotropic effect by relaxing smooth muscle) and the workload of the heart, thus decreasing the need for oxygen.
It is also used for angina, dysrhythmias, or hypertension.
Should be used with caution in the client with congestive heart failure, bradycardia, or atrioventricular block.

Side effects of CCB:

Bradycardia, hypotension, reflex tachycardia because of hypotension, headache, dizziness and lightheadedness, fatigue, peripheral edema, constipation, flushing of the skin, changes in liver and kidney function

NURSING CONSIDERATION/ INTERVENTIONS OF CCB:

- Monitor vital signs
- Monitor for signs of heart failure
- Monitor liver enzyme level
- Monitor kidney function tests
- Instruct the client not to discontinue the medication.
- Instruct the client to notify the HCP if dizziness or fainting occurs.
- Instruct client not to crush or chew sustained-release tablets.

VASODILATORS MEDS

- HYDRALAZINE
- NITROGLYCERIN
- SODIUM NITROPRUSSIDE

Purpose: used to widen the blood vessels to increase the flow of blood and lower blood pressure.

Side effects/teaching:

Headaches, nausea, and dizziness (especially older people)
Teach clients not to drink grapefruit juice while taking this medication. May interact negatively with cold medicine.

DIURECTICS (WATER PILLS)

Amiloride, Hydrochlorothiazide

Thiazide, chlorthalidone

Purpose: used to lower blood pressure

Side effects

Frequent urination, dehydration, blurred vision, fatigue, rash, loss of appetite
Monitor blood pressure and kidney function.

LOOP DIURETICS MEDS

- Bumetanide (bumex)
- Ethacrynic (Edecrin)

- Furosemide (Lasix)
- Furosemide (Demadex)

Purpose: used for hypertension, pulmonary edema, edema associated with heart failure, hypercalcemia, and renal disease

- Common side effects of the loop diuretics includes:
- Dizziness
- Headache
- Gastrointestinal upset
- Hyponatremia
- Hypokalemia
- Dehydration

Tiredness

Nursing Consideration/CAUTIONS of loop diuretics

Avoid taking loop diuretics if you have certain conditions such as: hyperkalemia, severe hyponatremia, hypotension.

Oliguria

If you are expecting to have fluid depletion such as during surgery.

ANTIANXIETY/MINOR TRANQUILIZER MEDICATIONS (BENZODIAZEPINE)

- Alprazolam (Xanax)
- Lorazepam (Ativan)
- Clordiazepoxide (Librium)
- Diazepam (Valium)
- Clonazepam (Klonopin)
- Oxazepam (Serax)
- Prazepam (Centrax)
- Halazepam (Paxipam)

SIDE EFFECTS OF ANTIANXIETY MEDS:

- For all: dizziness,
- Poor concentration
- Impaired judgement
- Drowsiness
- Headache
- Dry mouth
- Muscle weakness
- Nausea
- Confusion

Side Effects of CLONAZEPAM (KLONOPIN)

Alertness

Side Effects of OXAZEPAM (SERAX)

Decreased blood pressure

Treatment Cause: For Diazepam and Clonazepam – Ensure you check the functionality of the following systems of the body before administration of medication.

- Cardiac (heart)
- Pulmonary (lungs)
- Renal (kidney)
- Hepatic (liver)

Treatment Causes for Oxazepam (Serax), Prazepam, and Halazepam

Please note daily doses are as follows:

- Oxazepam (Serax), 30–60 mg
- Prazepam 20–60 mg
- Halazepam 20–160 mg
- Alprazolam (Xanax) causes panic attacks.
- Lorazepam (Ativan) and Oxazepam (Serax) ensure safety with the elderly patients.

The nursing considerations/usual course of treatment of anxiety includes:

- Low starting dose
- Awareness of addiction potential
- To discontinue, ensure slow, gradual reduction in doses.

NON-BENZODIAZEPINE ANTIANXIETY AGENT

BUSPIRON HYDROCHLORIDE (BUSPAR): no addiction potential. It takes three weeks to work. Do not give medication as PRN. Less sedating than others.

ANTIDEPRESSANTS MEDICATIONS

TRICYCLICS (TCAs) – Typical Antidepressants

- Amitriptyline (Elavil)
- Desipramine (Norpramin)
- Imipramine (Tofranil)
- Nortriptyline (Aventyl, Pamelor)

SIDE EFFECTS:

- Dry mouth
- Constipation
- Difficulty voiding
- Blurred vision

- Cardiovascular difficulties
- Sedation
- Anxiety/restlessness
- Decrease seizure threshold
- Weight gain
- Anticholinergic crisis
- Contraindications:
- Glaucoma
- Prostate
- Pregnancy
- Alcohol

Nursing consideration/usual course of treatment of TCAs:

- History of success
- Low starting doses
- Gradual increase to one time daily
- HS dose most beneficial
- Two to three-week lag period
- Treatment six to twelve months
- Lifetime for some
- Check liver function test
- Over 40: EKG and cardiac history
- Highly toxic in excessive amounts
- It can be very suicidal; do not give entire week's supply.

ATYPICAL ANTIDEPRESANTS MEDICATIONS

BUPROPION (WELLBUTRIN, ZYBAN)

- DAILY DOSE 225–450 mg
- MIRTAZPINE (REMERON)
- Daily dose 14–45 mg
- TRAZODONE (DESYREL)
- Daily dose 150–400 mg

SIDE EFFECTS

- No weight gain or sexual dysfunction
- Headache
- Insomnia
- Restless
- Nausea
- Seizures

- Sedation
- Hypotension
- Weight gain
- GI disturbance
- Sexual dysfunction
- Tremors
- Not a first line drug
- Trazodone – side effects Priapism
- Dizziness
- Orthostatic hypotension

Nursing Consideration and Usual Course of Treatment of ATYPICAL ANTIDEPRESANTS Same as: TCAs, SSRI, and SNRI

MOOD STABILIZERS: ANTI-MANIC MEDICATIONS

1. LITHIUM CARBONATE

- LITHOBID
- ESKALOTH
- LITHONATE
- Daily dose ACUTE 1800 mg/day
- Maintenance 900–1200 mg/day
- SIDE EFFECTS:
- Mild 05–1.5 level
- Increased urination
- Loose stool
- Fatigue
- Swelling
- Poor concentration
- Thirst
- Tremors
- Nausea
- Weight gain
- Moderate 1.5–2.0 level
- Incoordination
- Coarse hand tremor
- GI upset (call the doctor)
- Mental confusion
- Muscle pain (call the doctor)
- Hyperirritability (call the doctor)
- Severe 2.0–2.5 level

- Serious EEG changes
- Ataxia/slurred speech
- Blurred vision
- Stupor
- Hypertension
- Cardiac arrhythmia
- Coma
- Death

NURSING CONSIDERATION AND USUAL TREATMENT OF LITHIUM

- Renal function
- Thyroid status
- R/O neurological disorders and pregnancy
- Take 10–14 days for antimanic effects: often given with antipsychotics
- Start does 900–1500 mg
- Slowly increase
- Blood levels three times per week until stable between 0.5–1.5
- Antibiotics and nonsteroidal anti-inflammatory agents (NSAIDs) increase lithium level.
Caffeine can lower level.
- Maintain regular salt intake and fluids. No diuretics. (no Lasix)
- Give with meal.
- Hold dose and contact doctor if:
- Increased side effects
- High lab results
- Fluid loss

2. CARBAMAZEPINE

- TEGRETOL
- Daily dose 800–1200 mg/day
- SIDE EFFECTS -TREGRETOL
- Agranulocytosis
- Aplastic anemia
- Sedation

3. VALPROIC ACID 750–1000 mg/day
SIDE EFFECTS OF VALPROIC ACID

- Tremors:
- GI upset
- Weight gain
- Nursing Consideration and Usual Course Treatment OF VALPROIC ACID
- Liver function
- Cardiac function

- Contraindicated
- Bone marrow suppression
- Hypersensitivity to TCAs
- Begin low dose
- Follow blood levels for 6–8 weeks due to liver enzymes speeding its own metabolism.
- Look for diplopia, incoordination, and sedation, signaling high levels.
- Helpful with:
- Angry or dysphoric rapid cyclists
- Angry manic
- Dysphoric manic
- Poor response to lithium
- Same as Tegretol
- Check for signs of hepatitis.
- Fever
- Chills
- Pain upper right quadrant
- Dark urine
- Jaundice

4. CLONAZEPZM

- BENZODIAZEPINE (KLONOPIN)
- SIDE EFFECTS: Sedation – Ataxia and Incoordination.
- Usual course of treatment; helpful in psychomotor agitation
- 5. New drugs:
- LAMOTRIGINE (LAMICAL)
- GABAPETIN (NEURONTIN)
- SIDE EFFECTS:
- LAMOTRIGINE:
- Rash
- Headaches; ensure to rest and drink plenty of fluids
- Feeling drowsy, sleepy, or dizzy
- Aggression or feeling irritable or agitated
- Shaking tremor
- Difficulty sleeping
- Diarrhea
- Feeling or being sick (nausea or vomiting)
- GABAPETIN (NEURONTIN)
- Same as Lamotrigine and plus
- Mood changes
- Swollen arms and legs
- Blurred vision

- Dry mouth

Usual course of treatment: LAMOTRIGINE (LAMICAL) and GABAPETIN (NEURONTIN): Anticonvulsant is used in bipolar disorder.

DELECTIVE SEROTONIN REUPTAKE INHIBITORS (SSRIs)
FLUXETINE (PROZAC WEEKLY, PROZAC, SARAFEM)
CITALOPRAM (CELEXA)
SERTRAINE (ZOROFT)
PAROXETINE (PAXIL, PEXEVA, PAXIL CR)
ESCITALOPRAM (LEXAPRO)
SIDE EFFECTS:

- Insomnia
- Sexual dysfunction
- Fewer side effects than TCAs
- Low sedate
- Low anticholinergic side effects:
- Diarrhea, migraines, less weight gain
- Serotonin syndrome:
- May be life threatening
- Confusion
- Agitation
- Myoclonus
- Diarrhea

Nursing considerations and course of treatment of SSRIs:
Overall treatment is the same as TCA. If insomnia, give in a.m. only.
It takes one to three weeks lag period.
Watch out between two to five weeks before new drugs.
Serotonin syndrome
Stop drugs.
Anticonvulsants for seizure
Serotonin antagonist clonazepam

MONOAMINE OXIDASE INHIBITORS (MOAIs)
PHENELZINE (NARDIL)
TRANYLCYPROMINE (PARNATE)
ISOCARBOXAZID (MARPLAN)
SELEGILINE (EMSAM)
SIDE EFFECTS:

- Hypotension – Elderly

- Insomnia
- Weight gain
- Cardiac changes
- Contraindications:
- Cardiac problems
- Migraines
- Drugs
- Liver
- Pregnancy
- BP medication

Special Diet Restriction:

- Aged cheese
- Sour cream
- Chianti wine
- Beer, sherry, smoked dried foods
- Yeast products, yogurt
- Artificial sweetener
- Overripe foods, e.g., banana
- Fermented foods, e.g., pickle
- Fava beans, chocolate
- Caffeine in any food.

Hypertensive Crisis

- Severe headaches
- Stiff sore neck
- Flushing; cold, clammy skin
- Tachycardia
- Severe nose bleeds
- Pupils dilated
- Chest pain, stroke
- Coma, death

Nursing Intervention and Usual Course of Treatment

Begin tyramine restricted diet 48 hours before start.

Contraindications:

- Cold and allergy drugs, anesthesia, sedatives, stimulants, wear medical alert tag; ER – if severe headaches occur continue diet two weeks after discontinuing drugs.
- Wash out two to three weeks before starting new antidepressants.

Treatment for hypertensive crisis:

- Take vital signs.

- Nurse stays with patient
- Inform physician
- May use antihypertensive drugs to reduce BP, Regitine 5mg IV
- Antidote: Nitroprusside

SELECTIVE NOREPINEPHRINE REUPTAKE INHIBITORS (SNRI)

NEFAZODONE (SERZONE)

Daily dose 300–600 mg

VANLAFAXINE (EFFEXOR)

Daily dose 75–375 mg

Side Effects of SNRI

- Dizziness
- Dry mouth
- Somnolence
- Low sexual dysfunction
- Forty percent response rate when other drugs have failed
- Confusion
- Same side effects as Nefazodone (serzone)
- Plus, sweating
- Anorexia
- Sexual dysfunction

NURSING CONSIDERATION AND USUAL COURSE OF TREATMENT

History of success

- Low starting doses
- Gradual increase to one time daily
- HS dose most beneficial
- Two to three week lag period
- Treatment six to twelve months
- Lifetime for some
- Check liver function test.
- Over 40: EKG and cardiac history
- Highly toxic in excessive amounts
- It can be very suicidal; do not give an entire week's supply.

VANLAFAXINE (EFFEXOR) – also has same as TCAs, SSRI, and SNRI.

JACKS NCLEX REVIEW

PART 3

PEDIATRIC MEDICATION ADMINISTRATION AND CALCULATIONS

Children cannot swallow tablets, so most pediatric medications are liquids or suspensions.
To measure solutions, an oral plastic syringe or other acceptable measurement or administration device can be used, depending on the child's developmental age.
Caregivers should receive instructions from the health care provider on how to measure and administer pediatric medications.
Doses should always be double-checked to ensure accuracy. It is also important to store medication safely and out of reach of children.
Parents and caregivers should always read the label before administering medication.
When giving medication, it is important to be aware of possible side effects and to contact a health care provider with any questions or concerns.
Medication should be taken as prescribed and not be stopped or changed without consulting the health care provider first.
It is also important to monitor the child for any changes in behavior or health after taking the medication.
Finally, it is important to keep records of all medications given including the dosage, time, and date of administration.

Pediatrics Injection Sites:

- Vastus lateralis
- Rectus femoris
- Ventrogluteal
- Deltoid

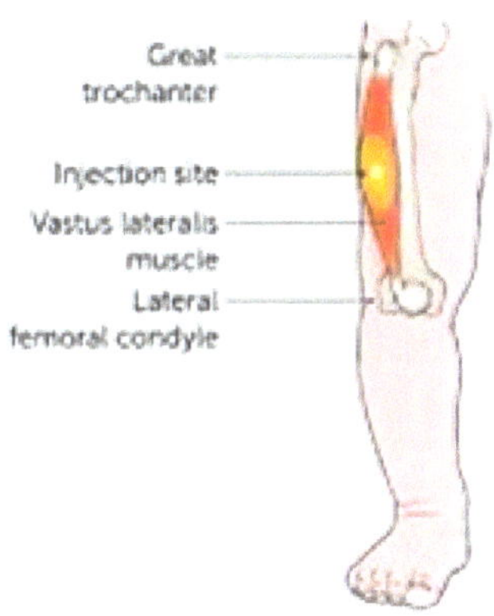

Conversion of Body Weight

Measurement:

1 lb. = 16 oz.
Lb. = 1 kg.
Pounds to Kilograms
2.2 lb. = 1 kg.
When converting from pounds to kilograms, divide by 2.2.
Kilograms are expressed to the nearest tenth.
Kilograms to pounds
1 kg. = 2.2 lb.
When converting from kilograms to pounds, multiply by 2.2. Pounds are expressed to the nearest tenth.

PRACTICE QUESTIONS

The nurse is providing medication instructions to a parent. Which statement by the parent indicates a **need for further instruction?**

1 "I should cuddle my child after giving the medication."
2 "I can give my child a frozen juice bar after he swallows the medication."
3 "I should mix the medication in the baby food and give it when I feed my child." Correct!
4 "If my child does not like the taste of the medicine, I should encourage him to pinch his nose and drink the medication through a straw."

Rationale: The nurse would teach the parent to avoid putting medications in foods because it may give an unpleasant taste to the food, and the child may refuse to accept the same food in the future. Also, the child may not consume the entire food served and as such may not receive the required medication dosage. The mother should provide comfort measures immediately after medication administration.

A pediatric client with ventricular septal defect repair is placed on a maintenance dosage of digoxin. The dosage is 8 mcg/kg/day, and the client's weight is 7.2 kg. The HCP prescribes the digoxin to be given twice daily. The nurse prepares how many mcg of digoxin to administer to the client at each dose?

1 12.6 mcg
2 21.4 mcg
3 28.8 mcg Correct!
4 32.2 mcg

Solution: Rationale calculate the daily dosage by weight first.
8 mcg / day x 7.2 kg = 57.6 mcg/ day
The HCP prescribes digoxin twice daily; two doses in 24 hours will be administered:
$\frac{57.6 \text{ mcg / day}}{2 \text{ doses}}$ = 28.8 mcg for each dose.

1. Signs of child abuse

- Injuries to the eyes or both sides of the head or body
- Regularly sustaining injuries such as bruises, cuts, and burns, grab marks, human bite marks, cigarette burns or impressions of other instruments.
- Destructive, aggressive or disruptive behavior
- Passive, withdrawn or emotionless behavior
- Fear of returning home or fear of the parent(s)

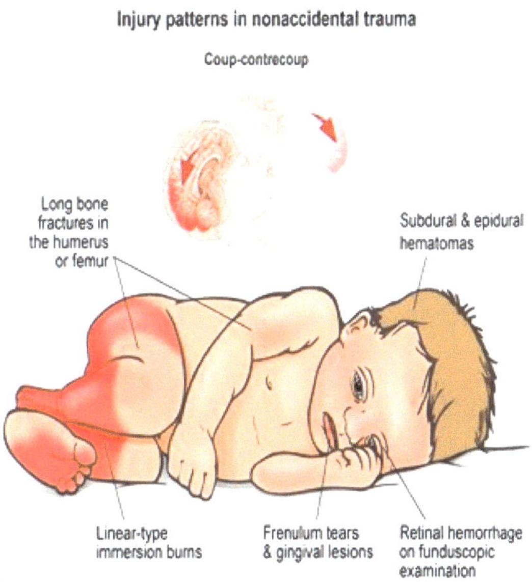

2. Injury patterns in nonaccidental trauma

They should be aware of signs of physical, sexual, and emotional abuse and comply with state or provincial mandatory reporting.
Shaken Baby Syndrome (irritability or lethargy, poor feeding, emesis, seizures)
Burns in the shape of household items, from cigarettes, or from immersion in scalding liquid
Repeated injuries in varied stages of healing (bruises, burns, fractures)
Injuries to the genitalia
Lapsed time between the injury and the time care is sought
Inconsistency between the injury and the caregiver's explanation of the injury (client's developmental stage, mechanism of injury)
Toddlers and young children are prone to many accidental injuries (aspiration or poisoning from foreign objects in the mouth, climbing onto and falling from furniture, pulling of objects from the table).
RN should instruct the caregivers on child safety measures within the home to prevent future injury.

3. ROOM ASSIGNMENTS

Remember that a client with an **active or suspected infection** should not be paired with a client who has a **fresh surgical wound or immunocompromised.**
A client with uncontained or excessive excretions, drainage, or secretions (profuse diarrhea, intractable diarrhea, draining wounds) is more likely to spread infection. If present, they should be assigned to a private room.

4. Suicide risks and assessment.
Risk factors for suicide include mental illness, substance abuse, and access to lethal means. It is important to assess a person's risk for suicide and provide appropriate interventions to reduce their risk. Professional help should be sought in cases where the person is at high risk for suicide.

Suicide risk & protective factors	
Risk factors	• Psychiatric disorders, prior suicide attempts • Hopelessness • Never married, divorced, separated • Living alone • Elderly white man • Unemployed or unskilled • Physical illness • Family history of suicide, family discord • Access to firearms • Substance abuse, impulsivity
Protective factors	• Social support/family connectedness • Pregnancy • Parenthood • Religion & participation in religious activities

Clients receiving treatment for depression and suicidal ideation must be carefully monitored for indications of increasing suicidal intent. The RN should assess:
Access to psychiatric medications
Availability of help during crisis (counselor, family)
Future goals and plans
Home and work environment risks
Overall affect and level of energy
Possible access to weapons
Clients who articulate long-term personal goals and family milestones are less likely to commit suicide.
Clients feel more energetic after beginning treatment, yet thoughts of suicide may not have fully resolved and the client may now have the energy to follow through suicide plans.

"No harm/no suicide" contracts are widely used in clinical practice to support a client's ability to avoid acting on suicidal thoughts. These agreements DO NOT GUARANTEE SAFETY AND ARE NOT THE BEST INDICATOR OF DECREASED SUICIDE RISK.

5. ADVANCED DIRECTIVES

Outlines the client's choices for medical care (CPR, mechanical ventilation) ahead of time.
This allows the family and healthcare team to **follow the client's wishes** at the end of life, when the client may be unable to make choices known. ***With an (ad) in place, the client's wishes are followed, even if they conflict with the wishes of loved ones.**

6. RN'S must ADVOCATE:

for client's wishes, even if family members are in disagreement.
must also consider applicable laws, regulations, and ethical codes
They must prioritize the client's aims and interests and respect all parties involved.
It is imperative to document all interactions to ensure client wishes are followed.
It is also important to remain impartial and professional in all client interactions. Additionally, it is important to ensure that all agreements are legally binding and that all parties understand the implications of the agreements.
This protects both the client and the company in disputes.
It is also imperative to maintain accurate records of all client interactions and agreements. This will ensure that any issues can be resolved quickly and efficiently.

7. Steps for male indwelling catheter insertion

- Perform hand hygiene and apply sterile glove
- Place fenestrated draped with shiny side down
- Use nondominant hand to grab penis below glens
- Use dominant hand to clean meatus with cotton ball or swab sticks
- Use dominant hand to insert catheter until urine return is observed
- Advance catheter to tubing bifurcation and inflate ballons.

1) Clean the insertion site with soap and water.

2) Lubricate the catheter insertion site with sterile lubrication.

3) Insert the catheter into the urethra, holding it straight.

4) Secure the catheter with a sterile dressing.

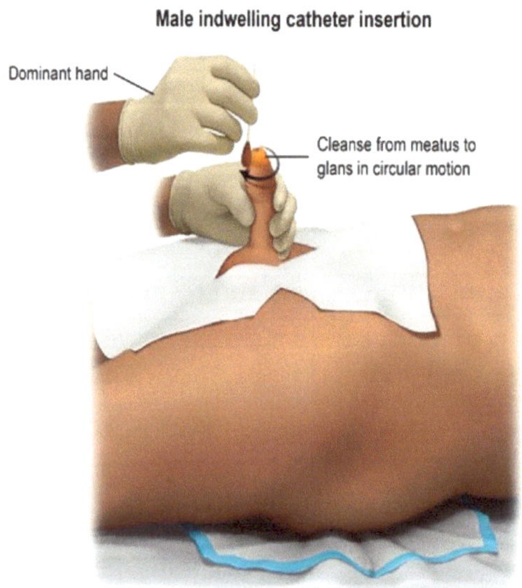

INSERT CATHETER TO BIFURCATION

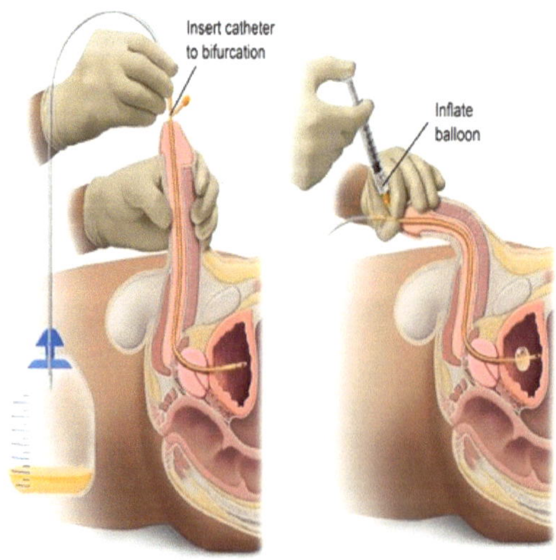

Steps for indwelling urinary catheter insertion for the male client include:

1. **Perform hand hygiene**, open sterile catheterization kit, and **apply sterile gloves** from kit **(Option 2)**
2. Maintaining sterility of gloves, **place sterile fenestrated drape** with opening centered over penis **(Option 3)**
3. Arrange remaining kit supplies on sterile field. Remove protective covering from catheter, lubricate catheter tip, and pour antiseptic solution over cotton balls or swab sticks
4. Firmly **grasp penis with nondominant hand**, retracting foreskin if present **(Option 6)**. Nondominant hand is now considered **contaminated** and remains in this position for duration of procedure.
5. Use dominant (sterile) hand to **cleanse** in a circular motion from the **meatus to the glans** with antiseptic solution using cotton balls or swab sticks **(Option 4)**. Use new cotton ball/swab stick with each swipe
6. Use dominant hand to pick up catheter and insert it until **urine return is visualized** in catheter tubing **(Option 5)**
7. **Advance to bifurcation** of catheter tubing. Hold in place and **inflate balloon (Option 1)**. Urine return in catheter tubing may be from urethra and does not indicate that balloon tip is fully inside bladder. Because male urethra varies in length, balloon should not be inflated until catheter is **fully advanced**.

Educational objective:
To insert an indwelling urinary catheter in a male client, perform hand hygiene, apply sterile gloves, place fenestrated drape, arrange

This ensures that the catheter has reached the bladder when it is inserted to the bifurcation of the Y. When the balloon is inflated before the catheter is inserted into the bifurcation, the urethra will be damaged and hematuria will result.

Bone healing
Depends on multiple factors (**nutrition, adequate circulation, and age**)
HEAVY ALCOHOL USE is associated with inadequate nutrition and can **DECREASE OSTEOBLASTIC ACTIVITY (BONE FORMATION)**

8. Pressure injury staging.

Stage	Clinical features	Illustration
1	• Intact skin • Non-blanchable with localized redness	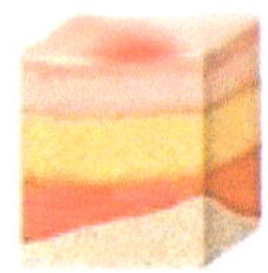
2	• Shallow, open ulcer • Red-pink wound with no sloughing • Possible intact or ruptured blister	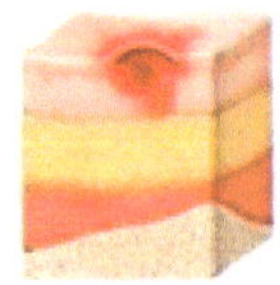
3	• Full-thickness skin loss with possible visible subcutaneous fat • No exposed bone, tendon, or muscles	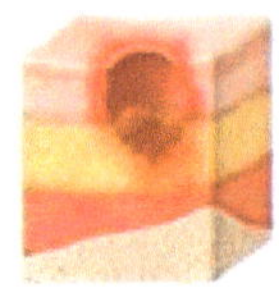
4	• Full-thickness skin loss • Exposed bone, tendon, or muscle	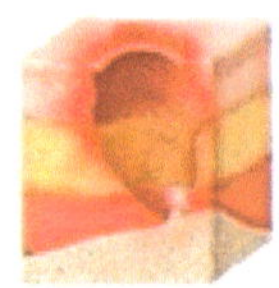
Unstageable	• Full-thickness skin loss • Ulcer base covered by slough and/or eschar that needs removal to stage	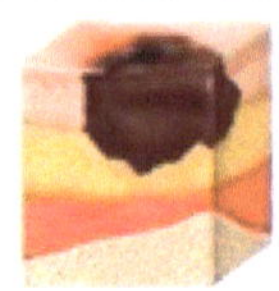

Stage 1: erythema of the skin.
Stage 2: Erythema with the loss of partial skin thickness including epidermis and part of the superficial dermis.
Stage 3: full thickness ulcer that involves subcutaneous fat.
Stage 4: full thickness ulcer with muscle or bone involvement.

9. Insulin Preparation

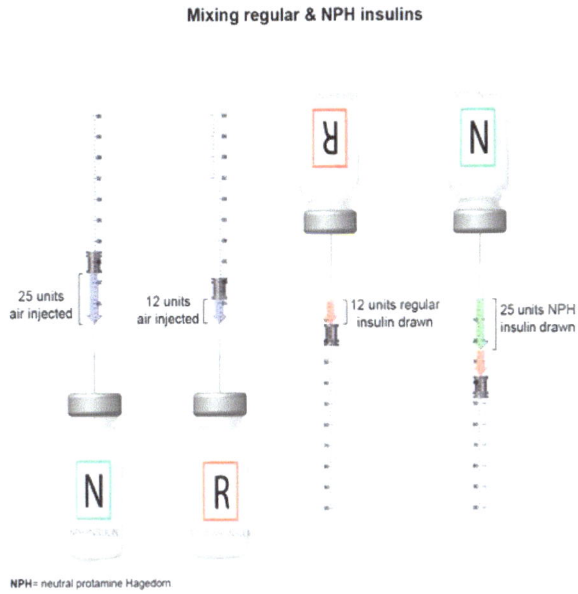

Intermediate acting insulins (NPH) can be safely mixed with short acting (regular) and rapid acting (lispro, aspart) insulins in one syringe.

10. Maslow Hierarchy of Needs

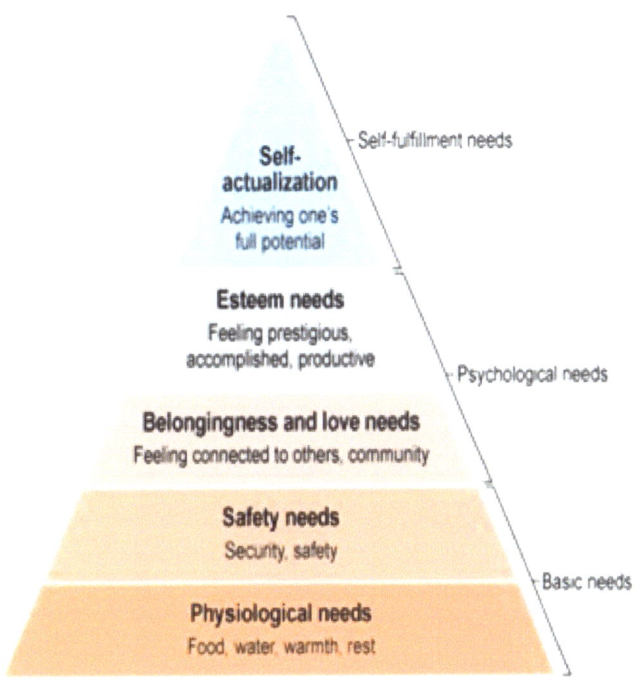

There are several different types of needs in the hierarchy, such as physiological needs (food and clothing), safety needs (job security), love and belonging needs (friendships), esteem, and self-actualization needs, which are listed in the order of importance.
The safety of the home environment is based on Maslow's hierarchy of needs.

11. LEAD POISONING

Houses built before 1978 have a high probability of containing lead-based paint. Active renovations can significantly increase the amount of lead released into the home environment, causing lead poisoning.

12. CHEST TUBE

Chest tubes are medical devices used to remove air or fluid from the pleural space. They are inserted through the chest wall and into the pleural space to drain out air or fluid. Chest tubes are often used to treat collapsed lungs or infections.
The chest tube is usually connected to a drainage system, which collects the air or fluid and allows it to be monitored. Chest tubes must be regularly monitored and should be removed when the drainage is minimal. They are usually removed in a few days or weeks.

Drainage collection chamber

The drainage collection chamber is located where the chest tube from the client connects to the system.
Drainage from the tube drains into and collects in a series of calibrated columns in this chamber.

Water Seal Chamber

Water seal chambers are used to create a hermetic seal around a device or system to prevent the entry of moisture or other contaminants.
They are commonly used in medical and industrial applications, as well as in sealants and waterproofing products.
Water seal chambers can also be used to maintain a certain pressure balance within a device or system. This is especially important when dealing with sensitive electronic components or hazardous materials.
They can also be used to detect leaks in the system. Water seal chambers are used to protect equipment from water, dust, and other environmental contaminants.
They can also be used to prevent the escape of hazardous gases or liquids from a system.
Excessive bubbling indicates an air leak in the chest tube system.

Suction control chamber (not vigorous)

The suction control chamber is a device used to regulate the suction pressure of a vacuum system. It works by controlling the flow of air using valves and dampers. This helps to ensure that the system operates at optimal levels of efficiency and safety.

Gentle bubbling in this chamber indicates that there is suction and does not indicate that air is escaping from the pleural space.

Dry suction system

Dry suction systems use compressed air to create a vacuum that allows for the removal of dust and other particles from a variety of surfaces.

These systems are often used in industrial settings to keep working areas clean and safe.

They are also used in medical settings for the removal of bodily fluids.

Dry suction systems are easy to operate and require minimal maintenance.

They are also cost-effective and can be used for a variety of cleaning and suctioning needs.

If the client has a known pneumothorax, intermittent bubbling in the water seal chamber is expected as air is drained from the chest, but continuous bubbling indicates an air leak in the system.

Notify the HCP if there is continuous bubbling in the water seal chamber.

NURSING INTERVENTIONS AFTER A CHEST TUDE INSERTION

An occlusive sterile dressing is maintained at the insertion site.

A chest radiograph assesses the position of the tube and determines whether the lung has re-expanded.

Assess respiratory status and auscultate lung sounds. Assess chest tube dressing for drainage and palpate surround tissue for crepitus.

Monitor for signs of extended pneumothorax or hemothorax.

Keep the drainage system below the level of the chest and tubes free of kinks, dependent loops, or other obstructions.

Ensure that all connections are secure.

Encourage coughing and deep breathing.

Change the client's position frequently to promote drainage and ventilation.

Do not strip or milk a chest tube unless specifically directed to do so by the HCP and if agency policy allows it.

Always keep a clamp and a sterile occlusive dressing at the bedside.

Never clamp a chest tube without a written prescription from the HCP; also determine agency policy for clamping a chest tube.

If the drainage system cracks or breaks, insert the chest tube into a bottle of sterile water, remove the cracked or broken system, and replace it with a new system.

Removing the chest tube: Based on the HCP preference, when the chest tube is removed, the client may be asked to take a deep breath and hold it, and bear down (Valsalva maneuver). A dry sterile dressing, petroleum gauze dressing, or Telfa dressing is taped in place after removal of the chest tube.

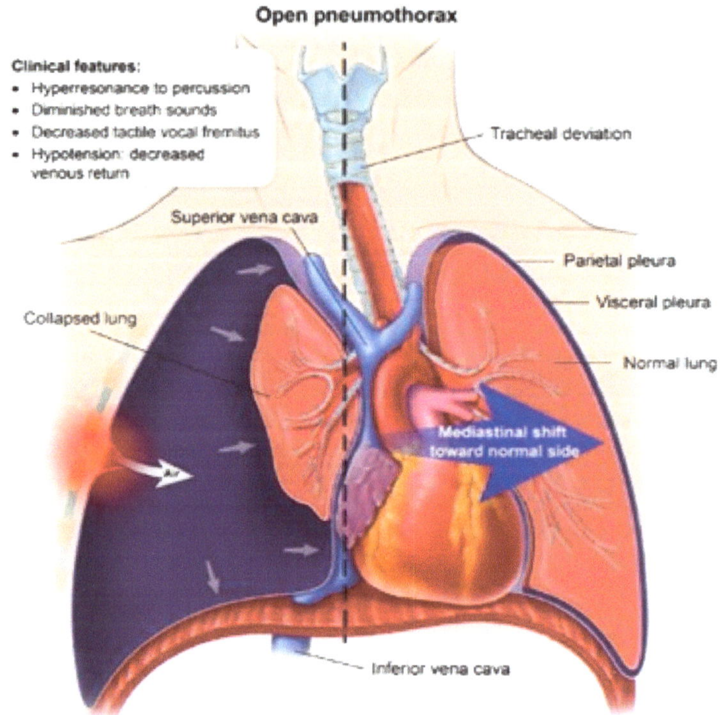

13. Ventricular trigeminy

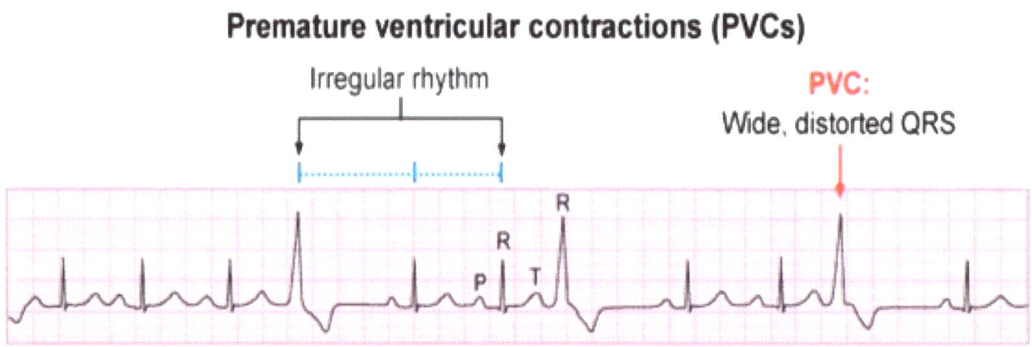

Premature Ventricular Contractions (PVCs) occur every third heartbeat which are exacerbated by hypoxia, electrolyte imbalances, emotional stress, stimulants, fever, and exercise.
Percutaneous coronary intervention and intracoronary stent placement via the femoral approach
Increased risk for retroperitoneal hemorrhage
Administration of antithrombotic drugs BEFORE, DURING, AND AFTER percutaneous coronary intervention (PCI) can **exacerbate potentially life-threatening bleeding from the femoral artery.**

Hypotension, back pain, flank ecchymosis (Grey Turner's sign), hematoma formation, and diminished distal pulses can be early signs of bleeding into the retroperitoneal space.

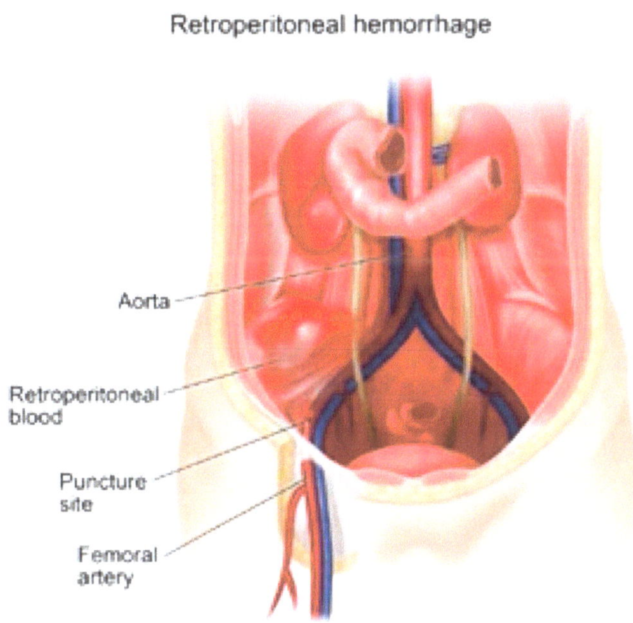

What are three signs of retroperitoneal Hemorrhage?
Assessment
Loin and/or abdominal pain
Often no cutaneous signs, but may have Cullen sign (umbilical ecchymosis) and grey turner sign (flank ecchymosis)
Plus, or minus palpable swelling
Hematuria
Hemodynamic instability and shock
Evidence of abdominal compartment syndrome (e.g. intra-abdominal hypertension, rental failure)

What is the most common cause of retroperitoneal hemorrhage?
Retroperitoneal bleeding is a serious illness that occurs when blood enters space in the back of the belly. This usually occurs after a traumatic injury and may require surgery to fix.

Symptoms of a retroperitoneal hemorrhage include abdominal pain, back pain, and dizziness. Other symptoms may include nausea, vomiting, and a rapid heart rate. It is important to seek medical attention if any of these symptoms occur. If left untreated, a retroperitoneal hemorrhage can be life-threatening.

Early diagnosis and treatment are essential for a successful outcome. Prompt medical care is necessary in these cases. Treatment may involve surgery, medications, and blood transfusions. It is important to take all prescribed medications and to follow up with a doctor regularly to ensure that the hemorrhage does not recur.

14. Disaster triage

Disaster Triage Color-coded Priority tagging	Characteristics	Examples
Emergent	Life-threatening injuries with high probability for survival if immediate treatment is received	• shock • Compromised airway • Unstable wounds • Chest trauma
Urgent	Serious injuries requiring treatment within 30 minutes and 2 hours	• Open fracture wound with palpable distal pulse • Large wounds
Nonurgent	Injuries requiring treatment but can wait for 2 hours or longer	• Infections • Minor burns or lacerations • Closed fractures
Expectant	Extensive injuries with poor prognosis regardless of treatment	• Pulselessness • Apnea • Severe neurological trauma. • Full thickness-burns. • >60% total body surface area.

During a mass casualty event the goal of the nurse is to triage rapidly and provide the greatest good for the greatest number of people. Clients are commonly triaged using a color-coded system and placed into four categories.

15. Sickle cell crisis

In the sickled state RBCs cannot carry enough O_2 from the lungs to the tissues, even with supplemental oxygen. **PRIORITY INTERVENTION: ADMINISTRATION OF IV FLUIDS TO REDUCE BLOOD VISCOSITY AND RESTORE PERFUSION TO THE AREAS AFFECTED BY VASOOCCLUSION**

Thromboembolic deterrent stockings (TED)

TEDs are specially designed socks that are used to reduce the risk of deep vein thrombosis (DVT). They are worn on the legs and lightly compress the veins, helping to increase circulation and reduce the risk of blood clots. TEDs are often recommended for long-distance travelers and those on bed rest.

16. Graduated compression stocking

Graduated Compression stockings are specially designed to apply pressure to the legs and feet to reduce swelling and improve circulation. They are often worn by people who suffer from conditions such as varicose veins or deep vein thrombosis. They are also commonly worn by athletes to increase blood flow and reduce fatigue.

Graduated compression stocking

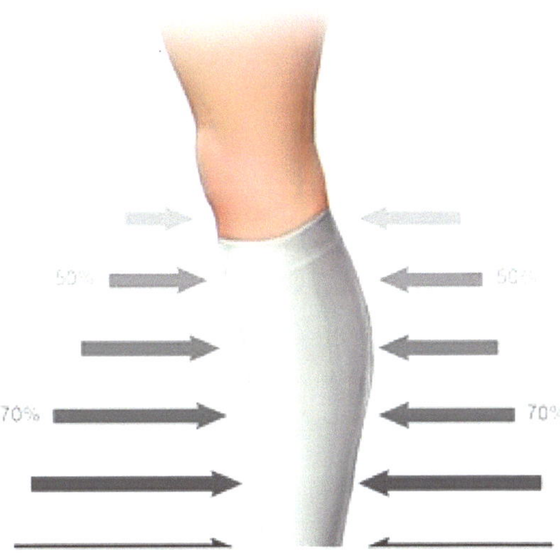

Elastic stockings provide graduated compression to the leg to promote venous return and reduce risk of venous thromboembolism.

RN should:

Select size of knee-length stockings by measuring length from the heel to the popliteal area and circumference at the widest point of the calf.

Ensure stockings are free of folds, rolls, or wrinkles as these may have a tourniquet-effect, exacerbating venous stasis and impairing perfusion.
Discrete wounds should be covered with occlusive dressings before application.
Stockings should be worn continually and may be removed one to three times a day for vascular assessment. Important to wear when legs are in a dependent position while sitting or standing usually during the day.

17. Basilar Skull fractures

Basilar skull fractures are a type of traumatic head injury. They occur when there is a force to the back or side of the head that causes the skull bones to break.
This type of fracture is often accompanied by other injuries, such as **traumatic brain injury or facial fractures**.
Common symptoms of basilar skull fractures include bleeding from the nose or ears, double vision, dizziness, headaches, and confusion. In some cases, the fracture can be life-threatening, and immediate medical attention is needed.

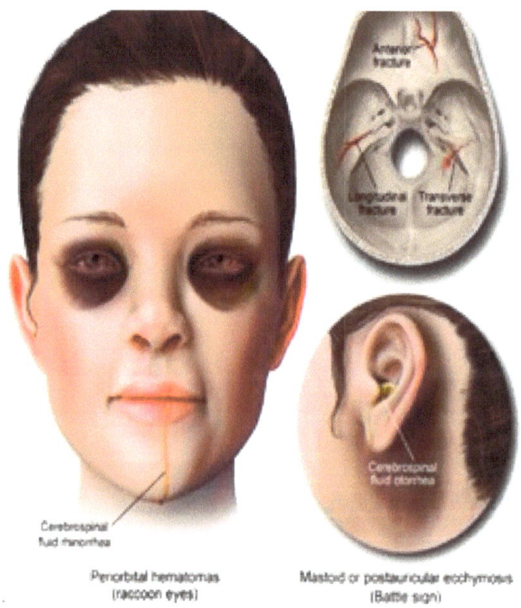

Poses a risk of serious intracranial injury, which is the most common cause of traumatic death in children due to its close proximity to the brainstem.
Requires immediate cervical spine immobilization, neurologic assessment, and airway, breathing, and circulation support.

18. Seizure Activity; PRIORITY: SAFETY!

Assist seated or standing clients to lie down while protecting the head, and position on the side to maintain a patent airway and prevent aspiration.
Losen restrictive clothing and clear the area near the client to prevent injury.

Administer oxygen as needed in response to signs of hypoxia.
Record and document the time and duration of the seizure.

19. Total Parenteral Nutrition (TPN)

Prescribed for clients with dysfunction of the GI tract.
Glucose is a primary component of TPN solutions; therefore, the nurse should monitor blood glucose and assess for **HYPERGLYCEMIA (polydipsia, polyuria, headaches, blurred vision)** Symptomatic clients should be assessed and treated immediately as hyperglycemia may lead to seizures, coma, or death.

Right task	• Within delegatee's scope of practice • Routine, frequently recurring task; minimal potential risk • Established sequence of steps; requires little to no modification for individual clients • Predictable outcome
Right circumstances	• Relatively stable client; noncomplex task • Adequate staffing, resources & supervision available
Right person	• Delegator should assess competency prior to delegating • Delegatee must have the appropriate knowledge, skills & abilities
Right direction/ communication	• Delegator needs to provide clear instructions; must include specific client concerns & observations to be reported back or recorded • Delegatee should verbalize understanding & have the opportunity to ask questions
Right supervision/ evaluation	• Monitor, evaluate & intervene as needed • Delegator retains ultimate accountability for task

21. Anti-psychotic side effects

Important antipsychotic side effects	
Extrapyramidal side effects	• Acute dystonic reaction: Sudden-onset, sustained muscle contractions • Akathisia: Subjective restlessness with inability to sit still • Drug-induced parkinsonism: Tremor, rigidity, bradykinesia, masked facies
Tardive dyskinesia	• Involuntary movements after chronic use (eg, lip smacking, choreoathetoid movements)
Neuroleptic malignant syndrome	• Fever, rigidity, mental status changes, autonomic instability

Atypical (second-generation) **antipsychotic** medications (eg, risperidone [Risperdal], quetiapine [Seroquel], olanzapine [Zyprexa]) are used in the treatment of **schizophrenia**, bipolar disorder, and other mental health disorders. The nurse should teach clients and caregivers about potential **side effects** of antipsychotic medications. Key teaching points include:

- dry mouth
- dizziness

- weight gain that can lead to diabetes
- blurred vision
- movement effects (for example, tremor, stiffness, agitation)
- sedation (for example causing sleepiness or low energy)
- loss of menstrual periods in women
- fluid retention
- dry mouth
- sexual problems
- headaches.

- **Extrapyramidal symptoms** (EPS) include akathisia (restlessness, fidgeting) and Parkinsonism (tremors, shuffling gait) **(Option 4)**. These specific symptoms are important to watch for, as EPS is easily mistaken for agitation or negative schizophrenic symptoms.
- Fever and muscle rigidity may indicate neuroleptic malignant syndrome, a potentially fatal condition requiring emergent intervention **(Option 1)**.
- Clients may experience **anticholinergic effects** (eg, dry mouth, constipation).
- Clients should change positions slowly to prevent **orthostatic hypotension (Option 2)**.

Other side effects: anticholinergic, orthostatic hypotension, sedation
Some HCP may prescribe medications to treat Extrapyramidal Side effect (EPS) (diphenhydramine, benzodiazepines)

22. Neuroleptic Malignant Syndrome

Neuroleptic Malignant Syndrome is a rare, life-threatening complication of antipsychotic medications.
Symptoms include muscle rigidity, fever, and mental status changes.
Treatment involves discontinuing medication and supportive care.
It is imperative to recognize the signs of Neuroleptic Malignant Syndrome early as prompt treatment is essential for an optimal outcome.
If left untreated, it can lead to permanent disability or death.
Patients should be closely monitored for signs and symptoms of this condition.
Potentially fatal condition requiring immediate intervention.

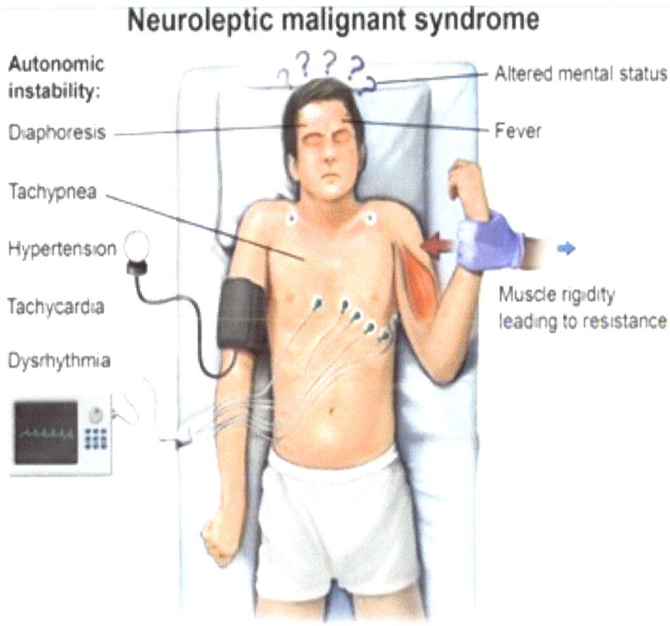

23. Blood products

Should not be left at room temperature for more than thirty minutes before a transfusion is started (increases likelihood of bacterial growth).

- The following are critical steps to follow before blood transfusion:
- Find the Current Type and Crossmatch.
- Obtain Informed Consent and a Health History
- Obtain Large-bore Intravenous Access.
- Assemble the supplies.
- Obtain baseline vital signs.
- Obtain blood from the Blood Bank.
- Blood transfusion reaction
- Fever
- Shortness of breath
- Chills
- Unusual itching
- Chest or back pain

A sense of uneasinessThe nurse should inform the patient to report any of the above reaction during and after blood transfusion.

24. Urosepsis

Bloodstream infection originating from the urinary tract.

INITIAL TREATMENT: MANAGEMENT OR PREVENTION OF SEPTIC SHOCK BY FLUID RESUSCITATION AND IV BROAD SPECTRUM ANTIBIOTICS. Broad spectrum antibiotics play a crucial role in managing septic shock by targeting a wide range of bacteria that may be causing the infection. These antibiotics are able to cover a broad spectrum of pathogens, giving a higher chance of effectively treating the infection before it worsens.

Chronic Kidney Disease (CKD) impairs the excretion of excess potassium. **ACE inhibitors (Lisinopril, Ramipril) or Angiotensin II receptor blockers (valsartan, irbesartan, losartan) can be used to manage hypertension secondary to renal disease; however, these drugs can worsen hyperkalemia.**

25. Colostomy

The opening creates a passage from the large intestine to the outside of your body. The opening, known as the anus, plays a crucial role in waste elimination. It allows the expulsion of solid waste, or feces, from the body, ensuring the removal of toxins and maintaining overall health and well-being. Stomach gas and solid stool leave the body through the stoma instead of passing through the rectum.

Appliances should be changed every **five to ten days** to prevent peristomal skin irritation.

Semi-liquid consistency of the stool from an ascending colostomy results in increased fluid loss.

INTERVENTION: DRINK PLENTY OF FLUIDS TO PREVENT DEHYDRATION

Decrease intake of gas-forming food (beans, onions, broccoli)

- In order to keep our bodies properly hydrated, we should drink plenty of fluids and consume foods with high water content, such as fruits and vegetables. Drink six to eight glasses of fluid a day to stay hydrated. (This amount includes both food and beverages containing water).
- There are several body functions that require water, such as digestion, absorption, and circulation. Fatigue, headaches, and dizziness can be caused by dehydration.
- To maintain good health, it is crucial to stay hydrated throughout the day.

26. Fall risk precautions and risk factors

- Fall risk precautions
- Fall risk precautions should include the use of guardrails, bed alarms, and other safety devices to reduce the risk of falls.
- Regular assessments should be conducted to identify any potential hazards and corrective action should be taken promptly to reduce the risk of falls.
- Regular exercise should also be encouraged to improve balance and strength.

- We strive to ensure that our clients are always safe. We take all necessary precautions to ensure their security, such as conducting background checks on all employees and regularly monitoring our premises. We also have a strict zero-tolerance policy for any form of violence or harassment.

Fall risk precautions

Fall risk precautions	
Standard	• Orientation to room & call light • Call light within reach • Bed in lowest position • Uncluttered room • Nonslip socks or shoes • Well-lit room • Belongings within reach
High fall risk	• Bed alarm • High fall risk signs • Room close to nurses' station • Color-coded socks & wristbands

- Promotes client safety

Fall risk factors

- Should be identified and addressed
- Any necessary safety equipment should be provided and used in accordance with safety regulations.
- Regular training should also be provided to keep employees informed on safety protocols.
- Lastly, it's important to have a system in place to investigate any accidents and near-misses, and to take corrective action to prevent future incidents. All these measures should be implemented to ensure the safety of employees.

Fall risk factors	
Age	• Age ≥60; ≥80 highest risk
History	• Recent previous fall
Elimination	• Bowel or bladder incontinence • Urgency or frequency
Medication	• Sedatives, opioids • Diuretics, laxatives • Antihypertensives • Central nervous system agents
Physiological	• Unsteady gait, dizziness • Weakness, limited mobility • Hypotension • Visual or auditory impairment
Cognition	• Altered mental status • Dementia
Equipment	• Lines, tubes, drains • Monitoring equipment • Sequential compression sleeves • Restraints

27. Preeclampsia, also called Toxemia: a potentially dangerous pregnancy complication characterized by high blood pressure. Pre-eclampsia usually begins after twenty weeks of pregnancy in a woman whose blood pressure had been normal. It can lead to serious, even fatal, complications for both mother and baby.

Main Causes

Pre-eclampsia is thought to be caused by the placenta not developing properly due to a problem with the blood vessels supplying it. Also lack of blood flow to the uterus could play a role.

Problem with placenta

Not enough nutrients

Inherited changes in genes

Having an existing medical problem such as diabetes, kidney disease, HBP, lupus or antiphospholipid

Previously having pre-eclampsia

Family history of the condition

You are over the age of forty.

It has been at least ten years since last pregnancy.

You were obese at the start of your pregnancy.

You are expecting twins or more babies.

PREECLAMPSIA (CONTINUED)

Definition	• New onset of hypertension & proteinuria or end-organ dysfunction after 20 weeks gestation
Hypertension	• Systolic BP ≥140 mm Hg or diastolic BP ≥90 mm Hg on 2 occasions at least **4 hours apart** **OR** • Systolic BP ≥160 mm Hg or diastolic BP ≥110 mm Hg confirmed on repeat check
Proteinuria	• ≥300 mg (0.3 g) of protein in 24-hour urine collection **OR** • Protein to creatinine ratio of 0.3 **OR** • Urine dipstick 1+ (when above not available)
End-organ dysfunction	• Thrombocytopenia (<100,000/mm^3 [100 × 10^9/L]) • Renal insufficiency (serum creatinine >1.1 mg/dL [97 mmol/L] or doubling creatinine) • Impaired liver function (ALT & AST twice normal) • Pulmonary edema • Cerebral or visual symptoms

COMPLICATIONS OF PREECLEMPSIA MAY INCLUDE:

- Fetal growth restriction. Preeclampsia affects the arteries carrying blood to the placenta.
- Preterm birth
- Placenta abruption
- Hemolysis elevated liver enzymes and low platelet count (HELLP) syndrome
- Eclampsia
- Other organ damage
- Cardiovascular disease

The ethical principles of beneficence, nonmaleficence, and standards in RN care dictate that a terminally ill client who desires a natural death should receive palliation, if desired, **EVEN IF CARDIAC AND PULMONARY FUNCTION ARE SUPPRESSED.** The nurse should always advocate for the patient's wishes.

28. Blood versus Amphotericin B

During Blood Transfussion, if the HCP prescribes Amphotericin B allow one hour between blood completion and starting of the drug to distinguish between transfusion-related or drug-related adverse effects. Amphotericin B is commonly associated with severe adverse effects including **hypotension, fever, chills, and renal toxicity, which is like the** Blood Transfussion reaction.

Amphotericin B is an antifungal medication used to treat serious fungal infections.
Blood is used to compare Amphotericin B effectiveness.
Amphotericin B is tested in laboratories by comparing its effectiveness to blood.
The results of the test can then be used to determine the medication's efficacy. The test results can also be used to identify potential side effects of the medication. Additionally, test results can be utilized to develop effective treatments or medications that are more effective and have fewer side effects.

Scope of practice		
RN	**LPN/LVN**	**UAP**
• Clinical assessment • Initial client education • Discharge education • Clinical judgment • Initiating blood transfusion	• Monitoring RN findings • Reinforcing education • Routine procedures (eg, catheterization) • Most medication administrations • Ostomy care • Tube patency & enteral feeding • Specific assessments*	• Activities of daily living • Hygiene • Linen change • Routine, stable vital signs • Documenting input/output • Positioning

LPN = licensed practical nurse; **LVN** = licensed vocational nurse; **RN** = registered nurse; **UAP** = unlicensed assistive personnel.

*Limited assessments (eg, lung sounds, bowel sounds, neurovascular checks).

End-Organ Dysfunction: A state of end organ damage occurs when a major body organ is severely impaired as a result of high blood pressure, low blood pressure, or low blood volume. The condition may manifest in the form of a heart attack, heart failure, pneumonia, stroke, or acute renal failure.
Thrombocytopenia (<100,000/mm^3[100 x 10^9/L])
Renal insufficiency (serum creatinine >1.1 mg/Dl [97 mmol/L] or doubling creatinine)
Impaired liver function (ALT and AST twice normal)
Pulmonary edema Fluid moves extravascularly into the interstitial space and alveoli of the lungs, causing pulmonary edema. It is possible to develop edema due to hydrostatic pressure, permeability, or mixed edema, which occurs when the membrane permeability increases along with the increase in hydrostatic pressure.
Cerebral or visual symptoms
The causes of cerebral visual impairment (also known as cortical visual impairment or CVI) may be caused by damage to the parts of the brain that process vision. CVI can be caused by a variety of fac-

tors, including brain injury, infection, stroke, or genetic disorders. These different types of damage can result in impaired visual processing, leading to difficulties with visual perception and interpretation

29. Ulcerative Colitis (UC) is a chronic disease characterized by inflammation and ulcerations in the large intestines, resulting in urgent, frequent, bloody diarrhea, abdominal pain, fever, and fatigue.

30. Autism Spectrum Disorder

Neurodevelopmental DO characterized by **impaired social interaction and behavior.**

Each child has unique communication needs.

Ease the child's anxiety and increase cooperation by:

Provide brief, concrete, and developmentally appropriate communication or demonstrations, explaining each step during procedure. ASD tends to be visually oriented.

Encourage caregivers to remain near the child to provide comfort and reassurance.

Reduce stimulation by limiting the number of staff members in the room.

Introduce staff or equipment slowly, preferably with caregivers nearby. This minimizes stress on the person with dementia. It also reduces the risk of changes in behavior. Lastly, it helps to create a sense of familiarity and routine.

Limit physical contact until conferring with the child's caregiver to assess which actions are soothing and which may trigger behavioral outbursts.

Potassium containing food

Foods highest & lowest in potassium		
	Foods highest in potassium	**Foods lowest in potassium**
Vegetables	Cruciferous vegetables, legumes, potatoes, green leafy vegetables, tomatoes, raw carrots	Asparagus, green beans, corn, cucumbers, okra, onions, green peas, green peppers
Fruits	Dried fruits, melons, avocados, oranges, mangos, nectarines, strawberries, bananas	Apple products, grapes, grapefruits, peaches, pears, pineapples
Dairy	Milk & milk products	Cottage cheese
Protein	Most fish & shellfish, most beef products, pork	Chicken, turkey, shrimp, tuna, eggs
Grains	Whole grains, granola, bran	Breads & pastas made with white flour, rice

Clients with **end-stage renal disease** are unable to excrete potassium; therefore, the nurse should teach them to **choose foods low in potassium** to maintain normal serum

Stroke

Sudden numbness or weakness in the face, arm, or leg, especially on one side of the body. Sudden confusion, trouble speaking, or difficulty understanding speech. Sudden trouble seeing in one or both eyes. Sudden trouble walking, dizziness, loss of balance, or lack of coordination.
Experiences cognitive dysfunction, neglect on one side, deficits in spatial perception, paralysis (hemiplegia) that increases risk for injury such as falls.

PRIORITY FOR STROKE PATIENT IS: SAFETY!

, neglect on one side, deficits in paralysis (hemiplegia) that increases risk for injury such as falls. Patients with ischemic stroke should receive intravenous thrombolytic therapy first.

A bolus of alteplase is injected intravenously, followed by an infusion over sixty minutes.

In order to treat an ischemic stroke, alteplase dissolves a blood clot that caused the stroke. Patients who receive it sooner have a better outcome.

Detecting and treating strokes early can minimize brain damage. Therefore, recognizing and responding to the symptoms of an ischemic stroke is essential.

Patients require physical therapy, occupational therapy, speech and language therapy, and psychological interventions to improve their quality of life.

The patient's family plays a crucial role in providing emotional and physical support. Caregivers and family members need to know the signs and symptoms of stroke and how to care.

They should also know the long-term effects of stroke and the different therapies available to the patient.

They should also know how to recognize signs of depression or anxiety and provide emotional support to the patient.

End Stage Renal Disease (ESRD) Overview. End-stage renal failure, also known as end-stage renal disease (ESRD), is the final, permanent stage of chronic kidney disease, where kidney function has declined to the point that the kidneys can no longer function on their own.
Patients are unable to excrete potassium; food low in potassium should be chosen.

Thrombolytic therapy (tissue plasminogen activator (tPA))

Dissolves blood clots and restore perfusion in clients with ischemic stroke.
Must be administered within a 3–4.5-hour window from onset of symptoms for full effectiveness.
Recent major surgery (within the past fourteen days) is contraindicated as it may disrupt the surgical site.

Loss of gag reflex and other major functions would most likely make the client candidate for TPA due to proof of deficits from stroke.
Thrombocytopenia <100,000 and/or coagulation disorders should not receive tPA as these conditions further increase the risk for bleeding.
Other contraindications: **hemorrhagic stroke, uncontrolled hypertension, and stroke or head trauma within the past three months.**

Lithium
Is a mood stabilizer most often used to treat bipolar affective DO
Narrow therapeutic index: 0.6-1.2 mEq/ L with many drugs interactions
Several medications can cause an increase in levels: thiazide diuretics, NSAID's, antidepressants.
Lithium can cause increase serum glucose levels; adjustment of antidiabetic meds is necessary.

Signs and symptoms of Lithium toxicity

- Dehydration, including dry mouth, fatigue and dizziness.
- Excessive thirst (polydipsia).
- Large urine output (polyuria).

Lithium toxicity	
Features	• **Acute:** Gastrointestinal findings - nausea, vomiting, diarrhea; neurologic findings occur later • **Chronic:** Neurologic - ataxia, sluggishness, confusion, agitation, neuromuscular excitability (coarse **tremor**)
Prevention	• Avoid sodium depletion; low sodium intake precipitates lithium toxicity • Eat regular diet & drink adequate fluids (2-3 L/day) • Therapeutic level is 0.6-1.2 mEq/L (0.6-1.2 mmol/L) • Level >1.5 mEq/L (1.5 mmol/L) is considered toxic

Developmental milestones of a preschooler (three to six years of age)
Manipulate small tools (scissors, pencils) to perform drawing and eating using utensils, gross motor activities like stair climbing.
They have a slow steady growth of extremities.
They increase their weight by three to five pounds yearly.
Height increases four to six cm yearly.
Toilet training is complete at this age
They undergo for vision 20/40 Snellen Test.
They may have "flat fee" at age threes.

Developmental milestones of preschoolers				
Age (years)	**Gross motor**	**Fine motor**	**Language**	**Social/cognitive**
3	• Walks up stairs with alternating feet • Pedals a tricycle • Jumps forward	• Draws a circle • Feeds self without help • Grips a crayon with fingers instead of fist	• 3- or 4-word sentences • Asks "why" questions • States own age	• Begins associative play • Toilet trained, except wiping
4	• Walks down stairs with alternating feet • Balances on 1 foot • Catches a ball	• Draws a square • Cuts with scissors • Ties a simple knot	• Names 2+ colors • Likes telling stories	• Begins imaginative/ group play • Recognizes analogies • Often focuses on self
5	• Skips • Walks backward • Uses a jump rope	• Draws a triangle • Ties shoelaces • Prints letters, numbers, or words	• Counts to 10 • Speaks full sentences • Names coins & days of the week	• Independently dresses & bathes • Identifies real from pretend

Abruptio Placentae

Vaginal bleeding and back or stomach pain.

Tenderness or rigidity may be felt in the stomach area.

The womb also experiences contractions, which are feelings of tightness and relaxation.

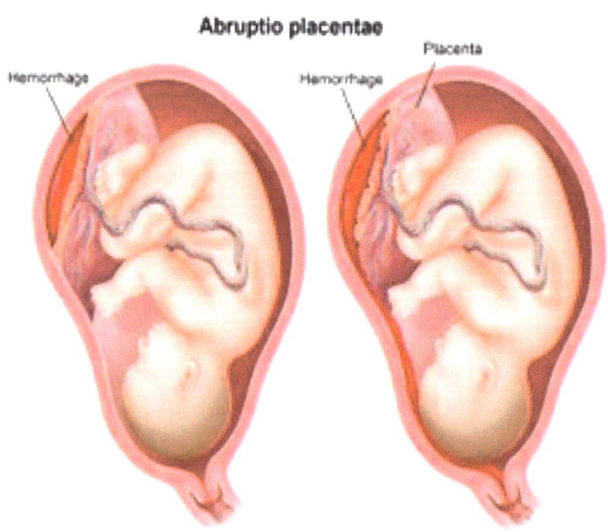

Concealed Bleeding   Visible Bleeding

Placenta prematurely detaches from the uterine wall.

Life-threatening complications can interrupt fetal oxygen supply and cause maternal hemorrhage
Signs/Symptoms: frequent contractions, abdominal pain, dark red vaginal bleeding, uterine tenderness, and elevated uterine resting tone.

PRIORITIES: Assessment of maternal vital signs, palpation of the abdomen/uterus, and continuous fetal heart rate monitoring

If with fetal distress/maternal hemodynamic compromise, prepare for emergency C-section.

*Vaginal birth is possible with a Mild or Partial **Abruption.**

ST-Segment Elevation Myocardial Infarction (STEMI)

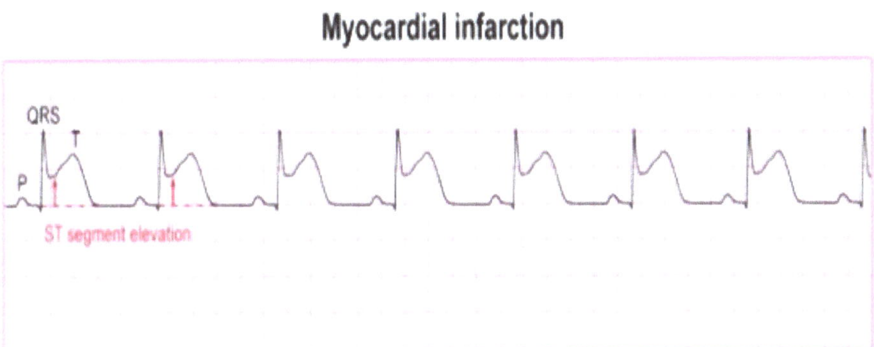

This is a dangerous heart attack or myocardial infarction that happens when an artery supplying blood to the heart suddenly becomes clogged or cannot pump enough blood to the rest of your body.

The nurse in the emergency department is assessing telemetry strips for assigned clients. Which client tracing is a **priority** for the nurse to assess?

1

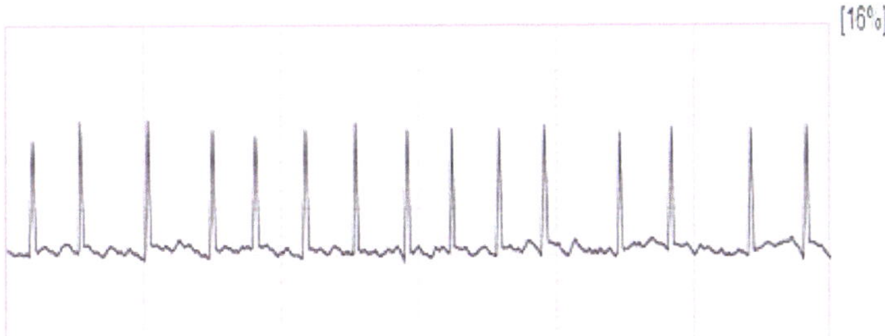

Atrial Fibrillation (AFib)

AFib stands for atrial fibrillation (AF), which is a type of arrhythmia, or abnormal heartbeat. AFib is caused by extremely fast and irregular beats from the upper chambers of the heart (usually more than 400 beats per minute). A normal, healthy heartbeat involves a regular contraction of the heart muscle.

Causes of Mechanical Ventilator Pressure Alarms

- Coughing
- Patient trying to speak.
- Exhalation before inspiratory flow stops.
- Kinks/bending in the ventilator circuit/biting circuit when on ET tube.
- Water in the ventilator circuit
- Increasing mucus or thick secretions blocking the airways.
- Inflammatory bronchospasm
- Symptoms of pulmonary edema
- Having a pneumothorax.
- Acute respiratory distress syndrome (ARDS).

Causes of mechanical ventilator pressure alarms

Location of problem	Causes of high-pressure limit alarm	Causes of low-pressure limit alarm
Ventilator circuit	• Kinked ventilator tubing • Condensation (water) in circuit tubing	• Tubing disconnect or leak
Endotracheal or tracheostomy tube	• Kinked endotracheal tube • Obstruction (secretions) in tube • Biting endotracheal tube	• Endotracheal or tracheostomy tube cuff leak
Client	• Increased airway resistance (eg, bronchospasm, excessive secretions) • Decreased lung compliance (eg, pneumothorax, atelectasis, pulmonary edema, acute respiratory distress syndrome) • Ventilator dyssynchrony (eg, anxiety, pain, coughing)	• Loss of airway (eg, total or partial extubation or decannulation)

Clostridium Difficile

Washing hands with soap and water is required to remove C. difficile spores; hand hygiene with foam or gel alone is ineffective.

History of Drug Abuse

Often requires a higher-dose analgesic or stronger opioid to achieve pain relief.
Contact the HCP to discuss client's frequent requests of Mo SO4 to alleviate uncontrolled pain.
ADMINISTRATION OF A PLACEBO OUTSIDE OF A CONSENTED RESEARCH TRIAL IS UNETHICAL AND DECEITFUL.

Pediculosis Pubis (pubic lice)

Pubic lice, also known as crab lice or crabs, are wingless, bloodsucking insects that can live and multiply on coarse hair, especially pubic hair. Hair in the armpits, eyelashes, eyebrows, or scalp can sometimes be affected, as well. Pubic lice infestation (pediculosis pubis) usually causes itching. Most often passed by sexual contact

Management:

Use lice treatment shampoo (1 percent permethrin) or rinse on pubic and body hair to kill lice!
After treatment, remove the nits with a fine-toothed nit comb, fingernails, or tweezers.
Wash and dry clothes, towels, and bedding with hot water and highest heat dryer setting.
Sexual partners should also receive pubic lice treatment.
All household members are at risk for developing pubic lice infestation and should be screened.

Witnessed collapse of a child

Children often develop respiratory distress and bradycardia before going into cardiac arrest. Rescue breathing for two minutes. If still <60bpm and there are signs of poor perfusion, CPR should be initiated.

Infants and children with a heart rate <60bpm with signs of poor perfusion are treated as pulseless.

Venous thromboembolism prophylaxis

Administration of anticoagulants
Application of compression devices
Frequent ambulation four to six times daily as tolerated
Foot and leg exercises
Avoidance of crossing legs and placing pillows behind the knees to elevate

Administering intermittent bolus feeding via NGT

Identify client using two identifiers.
Elevate the HOB 30–45 degrees before and thirty to sixty minutes after to minimize risk of aspiration.
Assess tube placement (tube placement marking, radiology report)
Assess bowel function (auscultate bowel sounds, check gastric residual volumes) before each intermittent feeding and medication administration.
Flush tube with 30 mL of water before and after intermittent feedings and medication administration to prevent clogging.
Administer prescribed feeding.
*Ensure that the feeding is not running fast or too cold to **avoid abdominal cramping.**

*Aspirated residual volume should be returned to the stomach to prevent metabolic alkalosis.

Preeclampsia with 3+ reflexes and two beats of clonus needs higher priority.

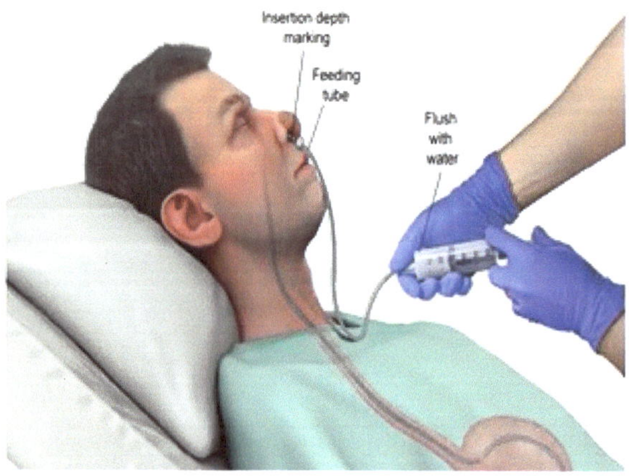

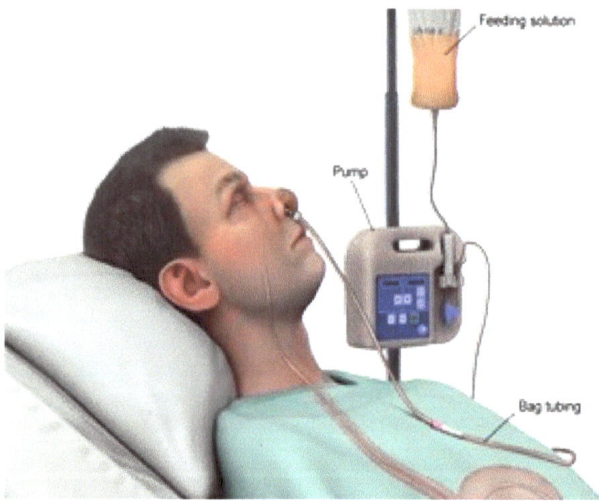

In case of clonus, a sustained beat of the foot (more than three beats) will result in an abnormal response.

There is a potential risk of seizures (eclampsia) due to this level of nervous system excitability.

It is a sign of seizure prophylaxis when it is present alongside other symptoms.

What does clonus indicate in preeclampsia?

An abdominal tenderness may be present in the right upper quadrant in pre-eclampsia due to hepatic swelling and capsular stretching. The condition of clonus is usually caused by severe pre-eclampsia because of neuromuscular irritability. Pre-eclampsia can also cause hyperreflexia, increased muscle tone, and uterine irritability. Additionally, the patient may experience headaches, blurred vision, and nausea.

How to assess clonus

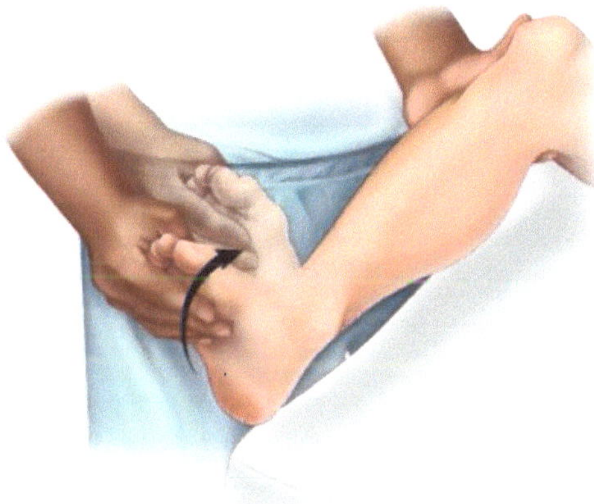

RN firmly dorsiflexes the foot with one hand while supporting the leg and ankle with the other hand. Abnormal finding results when rhythmic, jerking "beats" of the foot are present as the foot is released and allowed to fall back into plantar flexion.
Assessment of dark-skinned clients for petechiae is done in the conjunctiva of the eyes and the buccal mucosa because petechiae does not happen in the nail beds. Whilst cyanosis in dark-skinned clients is being checked in the nail beds, jaundice is being checked in the palms of the hands and the soles of the feet.

Chronic obstructive pulmonary disease (COPD), emphysema, chronic bronchitis
Emphysema- alveolar wall destruction; lung tissues lose elasticity (recoil) due to permanently enlarged "floppy" alveoli, which causes hyperinflation of the lungs (air trapping) as manifested by **HYPERRESONACE ON PERCUSSION AND PROLONGED EXPIRATION.**
Hyperinflation causes the patient to have a barrel-shaped chest.
Pursed-lip breathing (puffing), accessory muscle use, and tripod position are seen during exertion and as the disease progresses.

Arteriovenous graft
Surgical connection of an artery and a vein using a synthetic material to graft a hemodialysis access site
Postoperative infection of an AV graft may cause THROMBOSIS, GRAFT FAILUIRE, or SYSTEMIC INFECTION.
INTERVENTION: Immediately notify the HCP as this may require antibiotics and surgical removal of the graft.

Pregnant healthcare workers

TORCH (toxoplasmosis, other {parvovirus, varicella zoster}, Rubella, Cytomegalovirus, Herpes simplex virus) cases should not be assigned to a pregnant worker as these can cause fetal abnormalities. Furthermore, radiation exposure is also teratogenic and Zika virus should also be avoided contact.

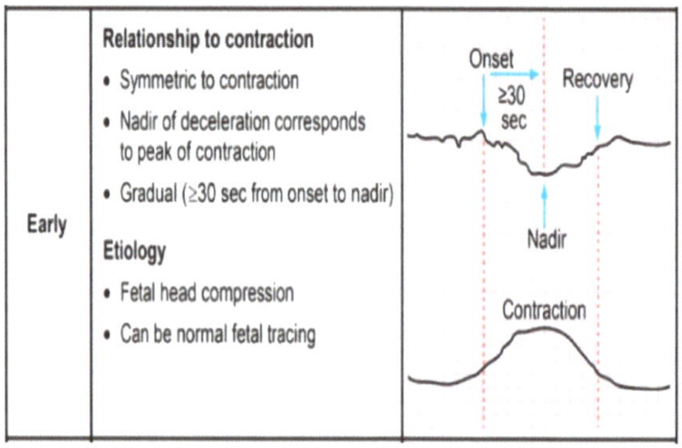

Early	**Relationship to contraction** • Symmetric to contraction • Nadir of deceleration corresponds to peak of contraction • Gradual (≥30 sec from onset to nadir) **Etiology** • Fetal head compression • Can be normal fetal tracing	

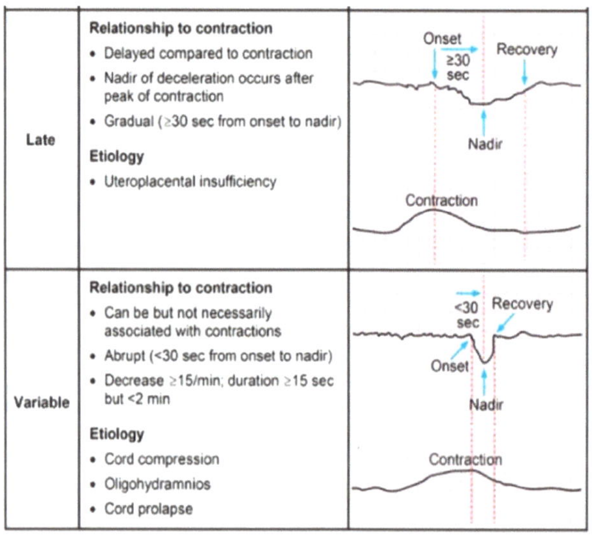

Late	**Relationship to contraction** • Delayed compared to contraction • Nadir of deceleration occurs after peak of contraction • Gradual (≥30 sec from onset to nadir) **Etiology** • Uteroplacental insufficiency	
Variable	**Relationship to contraction** • Can be but not necessarily associated with contractions • Abrupt (<30 sec from onset to nadir) • Decrease ≥15/min; duration ≥15 sec but <2 min **Etiology** • Cord compression • Oligohydramnios • Cord prolapse	

Contraction stress test evaluates fetal wellbeing under stress by identifying uteroplacental insufficiency. Uterine blood flow is decreased during uterine contractions, which stresses the fetus during labor. Negative tests have no late or variable decelerations and is associated with good fetal outcomes.

AED should be used as soon as it is available as early defibrillation is associated with improved CPR.

Move the client out of **LARGE BODIES OF WATER.**

Dry the chest area.

Removing transdermal medications patches and wiping chest of medication residue.

Entire body does not need to be completely dry to use the AED.

Increased intracranial pressure (ICP)

HOB: Thirty degrees to promote venous return from the head, which will decrease cerebral edema. Elevate instead of using pillows.
Keep the head and body midline and avoid extreme hip or neck flexion as this impedes venous drainage.
Administer stool softeners to prevent straining.
Keep the client in a calm environment with minimal noise and disturbances.
Suction only when needed to maintain airway and not longer than ten seconds.
Reduce metabolic demands. Treat fever aggressively but avoid shivering.

Respiratory Syncytial Virus

Common causes of respiratory infection and bronchiolitis in infants and children primarily during winter.
Affects the ciliated cells of the respiratory tract causing bronchiolar swelling and excessive mucus production.
INTERVENTIONS: (supportive)
Supplemental oxygen and suctioning
Elevating the HOB
Administer antipyretics
Initiating IV fluids
Contact isolation is required and droplet precautions if within three feet
Palivizumab (synagis) a monoclonal antibody is administered IM once monthly during the winter and spring to prevent RSV for children at high risk.

Parental refusal of necessary medication in a minor creates an ethical dilemma.
FIRST response:
ASSESSMENT OF A PARENTAL KNOWLEDGE DEFICIT regarding the client's condition.
ASK OPEN-ENDED questions.

Terminally ill patients in hospice set up often experience dyspnea (air hunger)

Reduce the perception of dyspnea by administering prescribed opioids to decrease respiratory effort, providing low-flow oxygen by nasal cannula, implementing comfort measures, and relieving anxiety.

Bipolar disorder

Manic clients demonstrate hyperactivity and distractibility and may refuse to sit long enough to drink or eat. RISK for: IMBALANCED **NUTRITION LESS THAN BODY REQUIREMENTS. (Physiological need according to Maslow) that takes priority over psychological, or self-fulfillment needs.**
PROVIDE: high caloric snacks and finger foods

Clients with multiple HCP and multiple prescriptions
Advised to bring all the medications they take regularly and occasionally to each appointment so that potential drug interactions can be evaluated.
Administer PRN medication for its prescribed purpose only.

Percutaneous Coronary Intervention
Overview: Percutaneous coronary intervention (PCI) is a non-surgical procedure used to treat the blockages in a coronary artery; it opens up narrowed or blocked sections of the artery, restoring blood flow to the heart.
Potential complications: **thrombosis, stent occlusion, bleeding/hematoma, and limb ischemia**
Immediately notify the HCP for **post procedure angina,** which indicates possible thrombosis or stent occlusion.

Constipated clients should avoid CAFFEINATED beverages as they promote diuresis and may lead to dehydration and worsening of constipation.

Physical Restraints
Perform **HOURLY NEUROVASCULAR CHECKS (**pulse, color, skin temperature, sensation, movement)
Briefly releasing restraints for skin integrity assessment and ROM every **TWO HOURS**
Offering fluids, nutrition, and toileting every two hours and as needed.
RN should regularly assess every hour the client's continued need for restraints.
Trial discontinuations are not permitted.

INFORMED CONSENT
The RN should ensure that the client meets the ff criteria: mentally competent adult; understand the procedure, risks, benefits, and alternatives; signs voluntarily without coercion.
A client questioning the need for a BT during surgery indicates an incomplete understanding of the risk and would invalidate the signature.
The client can provide informed consent once the effects of the sedating medications have worn off. (Hydrocodone duration of action is four to six hours.)

Tuberculin skin test reactions

Explanation

Tuberculin skin test reactions	
Response	**Consider positive in these clients/groups**
Induration of ≥ 5 mm	• HIV infected • Immunosuppressed (disease, medication) • Organ transplant recipients • Recent contact with person with TB
Induration of ≥ 10 mm	• Children age <4 or children & adolescents exposed to adults in high-risk groups • Injection drug user • Recent (<5 years) immigrant from high-prevalence country • Resident or employee in high-risk congregate area (homeless shelter, correctional facility, nursing home, health care facility)
Induration of ≥ 15 mm	• No known risk factors for TB

TB = tuberculosis.

Tuberculin purified protein derivative (PPD) skin tests (ie, Mantoux test) screen individuals for tuberculosis (TB) exposure. The skin is assessed at the bleb administration site 48-72 hours after

Latent tuberculosis infection & active pulmonary tuberculosis disease		
	Latent TB infection	**Active pulmonary TB disease**
Clinical manifestations	Asymptomatic	• Cough • Constitutional symptoms ○ Fever/chills, malaise ○ Weight loss, night sweats ○ Anorexia, fatigue
TB transmission	No	Yes
Diagnostic tests	• Positive tuberculin skin test & interferon-γ release assay • Normal chest x-ray • Negative sputum smear/culture	• Positive tuberculin skin test & interferon-γ release assay • Abnormal chest x-ray • Positive sputum smear/culture

TB = tuberculosis

Human Papilloma Virus
Common STD is often asymptomatic and may resolve spontaneously in young and healthy people.

HPV Vaccine
Teens and young adults less than twenty-six years old who have already become sexually active can benefit from HPV vaccine.

Pap Testing
Initiated at age twenty-one, regardless of sexual history.

67. Second degree AV block

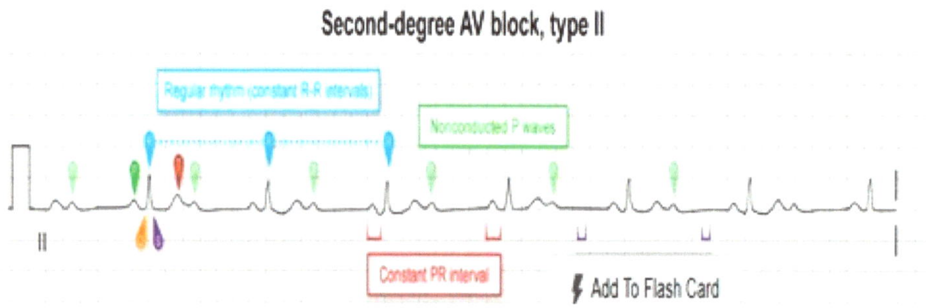

More p-waves than QRS complexes with dropped QRS complexes.
Can rapidly progress to complete heart block and is life-threatening
INTERVENTION: TCP and be prepared to pace the client if symptoms occur
Beta blockers can cause second degree heart block.

Caring for a client with a radial, brachial, or femoral catheter
Assess for: **HEMORRHAGE, INFECTION, THROMBUS FORMATIONS, AND CIRCULATORY AND NEUROVASCULAR IMPAIRMENT**

Sudden Infant Death Syndrome (SIDS)
Place the infant on the back to sleep on a firm surface and should not share a bed with anyone.
Avoid soft objects (stuffed toys, pillows). **NOTHING IN THE BED** with the infant is the best.
Avoid bumper pads for the crib.
Maintain a smoke-free environment.
Avoid overheating. Infants do not need an extra layer of clothing.
Breastfeed and ensure immunizations are updated.
Using a pacifier during sleep is appropriate but must be delayed until after breastfeeding is well established.
A sleeping sack "onesie" reduces the need for a blanket.

Initial Newborn assessments

Hypotonia: related to hypoxia, down syndrome, or a muscular/neurologic disorder
Sacral dimple: may be a sign of spina bifida occulta. A defect where the bones that protect the meninges and the spinal cord fail to close during gestation.
Single umbilical artery: associated with congenital defects particularly the kidneys and the heart
*Acrocyanosis: Cyanosis of the hands and feet are normal within seven days of birth.

Persecutory delusions (paranoid delusions) - believe that they are being persecuted or harmed.
Focusing on the client's feelings secondary to the delusion is an example of empathy that makes them feel that someone is trying to understand them and the nurse-client relationship grows.
Focusing on reality and verbally reinforcing it will decrease the time that the client spends thinking about the delusions.
Do not explore; it will make the client think more of the delusion.
Do not confront; it will hinder the development of a trusting relationship with the client.
Delusions are real despite proof otherwise. Do not present logical explanations to discredit the delusions.

HELLP syndrome (hemolysis, elevated liver enzymes, low platelet count)

Sever form of preeclampsia but hypertension may not be present.
Often mistaken for viral gastroenteritis due to its variable and nonspecific orientation
Sign/Symptom: **Right Upper Quadrant Pain Nausea/Vomiting, Malaise**
Severe complications: **placental abruption, lover failure, stroke, maternal/fetal death**

Irritable bowel syndrome

Dicyclomine (Bentyl): anticholinergic/antispasmodic to manage symptoms of intestinal hypermotility in clients with IBS (irritable bowel syndrome)
Contraindicated to clients with paralytic ileus.
Restrict gas-producing products (banana, cabbage, onions), caffeine, alcohol, fermented oligo-, di-, and monosaccharides and polyols (FODMAPS), honey, high-fructose corn syrup, wheat, and other GI Irritants (spices, hot/cold food/drink, dairy products, fatty foods)
Increase fiber intake (whole grains, legumes, nuts, fruits, vegetables), proteins, breads, bland foods.

Breast engorgement

For clients who choose not to breast feed, treatment focuses on managing symptoms while reducing milk production.
Apply ice packs to both breasts for fifteen to twenty minutes every three to four hours to reduce blood flow and swelling.
Applying chilled, fresh cabbage leaves to both breasts.

Taking an anti-inflammatory analgesic (ibuprofen) directed to reduce pain.
Maintaining firm breast support until milk flow is diminished.

TORCH infections

Toxoplasmosis, Other (Parvo B-19/ Varicella Zoster), Rubella, Cytomegalovirus, Herpes Simplex virus): Causes fetal abnormalities and should not be assigned to pregnant nurses

Donning and doffing PPE

Donning

Hand hygiene
Gown
Mask/respirator
Goggles/face shield
Gloves

Doffing

Gloves
Goggles/face shield
Gown
Mask/respirator
Handwashing

Preparing a medication from a glass ampule

The nurse breaks the ampule away from the body and discards it in the sharp's container.
Withdraws the medication using a filter needle to prevent injection of glass shards.
Avoids touching the needle to contaminate ampule edges.
Avoids injecting air to prevent spillage.

Separation or stranger anxiety (Pediatric)

This starts around six months and peaks at ten to eighteen months that can last up to three years of age.
It produces more stress than any other factors (pain, injury, and change in surroundings) for children in this age range. However, it is normal and resolves by age three years.
RN Interventions:
Adhere to the infant's home routine when possible.
Providing the favorite toy or pacifier
Encouraging caregivers to remain whenever possible during hospitalization.
Provide a quiet sleep environment with reduced stimulation to promote restful sleep.
Offering a familiar object (caregiver's shirt, blanket, voice recording) during stressful situations

Tension Pneumothorax

The client is experiencing a **second-degree type 2 atrioventricular (AV) block (Mobitz II)**, which is characterized by more P waves than QRS complexes. The **PR intervals are consistent** or constant, reflecting regular conduction of electrical impulses through the AV node, but **dropped QRS beats** randomly occur as ventricular conduction is blocked.

A second-degree type 2 AV block can **rapidly deteriorate** to complete heart block (third-degree AV block), which is **life-threatening**. The nurse should quickly obtain a **transcutaneous pacemaker**, assess the client for symptoms (eg, bradycardia, hypotension, syncope), and be prepared to pace the client if symptoms occur **(Option 2)**. If the client is asymptomatic, the pacemaker is kept nearby in case the rhythm deteriorates, and the health care provider is alerted.

(Option 1) A common complication following myocardial infarction is the development of new arrhythmias. Although a second-degree type 2 AV block is not completely unexpected in this client, it indicates a concerning situation that requires assessment and

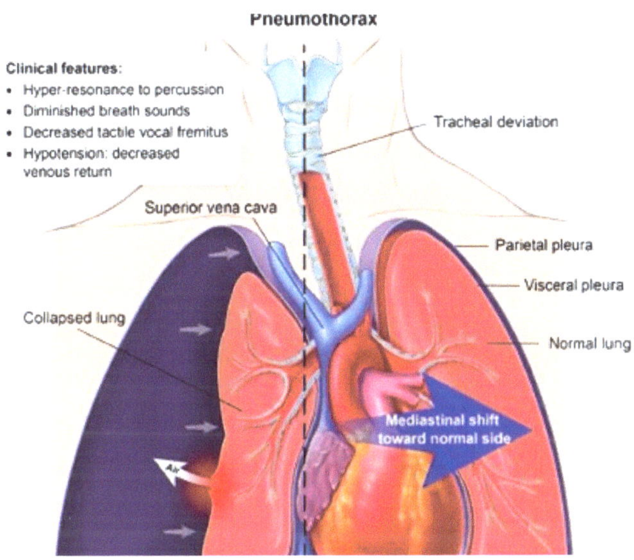

Tetralogy of Fallot (Pediatric)

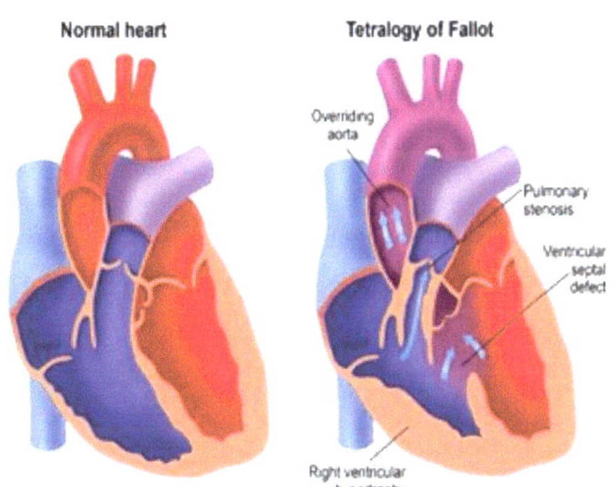

FOUR CHARACTERISTICS OF Tetralogy of Fallot (TOF):

1. **Ventricular Septal Defect (VSD):** Heart defects that affect the lower chambers of the heart. As there is a hole in the wall of the vessel, oxygen-rich blood and oxygen-poor blood can mix together, making it difficult for the body to obtain enough oxygen-rich blood.
2. **Pulmonary Stenosis**: In pulmonary stenosis, the pulmonary artery struggles to supply enough blood to the lungs due to narrowed or stiffened valves.
3. **Overriding of Aorta**: An overriding aorta indicates that the artery that carries oxygen-rich blood to the body is out of place and stretches across both ventricles. As a result, the body gets too much oxygen-poor blood.
4. **Right Ventricular Hypertrophy:** hypertrophy (enlargement) of the right ventricle: The right lower chamber of the heart is enlarged or thicker than normal, making it more difficult for blood to go through the pulmonary valve.

Sign and Symptom of TOF:
Cyanosis (88- 92 % oxygen saturation)
Clubbing – changes on the toenails and finger nails
Polycythemia – increase in the number of RBC in the body
Occurs in all states of chronic hypoxia
Increases oxygen-carrying capacity
Hyperviscosity increases risk of stroke and myocardial infarction (MI)
4.Failure to thrive (FTT)5. Tet spell: hypercyanotic episode that can happen when a child cries, becomes upset, or is feeding. INTERVENTION: Place the child in a knee-chest position (this reduces the volume of blood shunted through the overriding aorta and ventricular septal defect.)
Intervention for a child with tet/hypercyanotic spells:
Calm the child – place the child on knee to chest/ squatting position
Administer oxygen
Morphine
intravenous fluids
Neosynephrine
  IV administration
  systemic vasoconstriction
Opioid Medications (Mo So4) is considered if the dyspnea is not relieved by knee-chest position.

Cervical Cap Contraception
Used with spermicide (nonoxynol-9) applied inside the cap and a thin layer on the rim and the outer portion in the groove.

The cap should remain in place for at least six hours but no more than forty-eight hours after intercourse.
Use of cervical cap during menses or in the postpartum period increases the risk for toxic shock syndrome (TSS); an alternative contraceptive method should be used at this time.
Women with a history of TSS should not use cervical caps.

Type II Diabetes Mellitus

In Type 2 Diabetes Mellitus, the response to insulin is diminished, and this is defined as insulin resistance. During this state, insulin is ineffective and is initially countered by an increase in insulin production to maintain glucose homeostasis, but over time, insulin production decreases, resulting in T2DM.
Chronic hyperglycemia can cause microvascular damage in the retina leading to diabetic retinopathy, the most common cause of new blindness in adults.
A partial retinal detachment may be painless and cause symptoms such as curtain blocking part of the visual field, floaters, or lines, and sudden flashes of light.

Nitroglycerin administration procedures, storage, side effects

Tablets are heat and light sensitive (kept in a dark bottle). Opened bottles should be discarded after six months.
Take up to pills in a fifteen-minute period. Call EMS if pain does not improve or worsens after the first pill.
Avoid fatal drug interactions (erectile dysfunctions drugs: sildenafil, alpha blockers: terazosin, tamsulosin) is contraindicated and may cause lethal hypotension.
Headache and flushing may occur due to systemic vasodilation.

Trimethoprim- sulfamethoxazole (Bactrim)

Sulfonamide antibiotic (sulfa drug) used to treat bacterial infections such as UTI.
Glyburide is a **SULFONYLUREA** and has the potential to cause a sulfa cross sensitivity reaction.
Commonly used diuretics (thiazide, furosemide) are also sulfa derivatives.
Crystalluria is a potential adverse effect of sulfa meds and OFI should be at least two to three liters per day.

Cataract Surgery

Avoid activities that may increase IOP to decrease risk of damage to sutures or surgical site (bending, lifting more than five pounds, sneezing, coughing, rubbing, or placing pressure on the eye, straining during bowel movement)
Increase high fiber diet and advice OTC stool softener or laxative.
Educate that it may take one to two weeks before visual acuity is improved.
Common to experience itching like "sand" in the eye, photophobia, and mild pain for several days.

Purulent drainage, increase redness, and sever pain should be reported.
Advice to sleep on two pillows to decrease IOP.

Amoxicillin/Clavunate in liquid form
Shaken well before administration.
Use a calibrated measuring device.
Taken with or without food at evenly spaced intervals throughout the day to ensure therapeutic drug levels.
If nausea and diarrhea develop, administer with food.
Complete the full course of antibiotics even if the child feels better.

Albuterol: short term beta-adrenergic agonist (rescue inhaler)
Treats reversible airway obstruction associated with asthma.
Should not exceed two to four puffs every twenty minutes x 3 doses.
Sympathomimetic drug and mimic manifestations related to stimulation of the SNS that commonly include **insomnia, n/v, palpitations, mild tremor.**

Von Willebrand Disease
Genetic bleeding disorder caused by deficiency in Von Willebrand factor (vWF)
Intranasal desmopressin or topical therapies may be prescribed to stop minor bleeding.
TEACH: Patient to wear a medical identification bracelet
Notify HCP of signs of bleeding.
Use a humidifier or nasal spray to keep the mucosa moist.
Avoid aspirin and NSAIDS.
Avoid activities with high risk of injury like contact sports.
Maintain gum integrity by using soft-bristled toothbrush and gentle flossing.
Report heavy menstrual bleeding.

Clostridium difficile colitis is treated with metronidazole and vancomycin depending on severity and relapses.

Candida Albicans (yeast)
Causes infections of the vulvovaginal regions that often causes itching and painful urination due to urine stinging the inflamed area of the vulva.
Assessment: thick, white, curd-like vaginal discharge and reddened vulvar regions
Miconazole is an antifungal cream commonly prescribed for treatment using an applicator to the vagina.
BEST applied at NOC so it will remain for an extended period in the vagina.

Sexual intercourse is prohibited until the inflammation is resolved, usually three to seven days duration of treatment. However, sexual intercourse is not a significant cause of infection or reinfection, so partner evaluation is not needed.
Ensure proper hygiene of the perineum.
Wear loosely fitted cotton underwear and avoid synthetic garments.
Refrain from douching, which can introduce organisms higher up into the vaginal canal and cervix.

Handoff report inclusions
Client's name, location, age, gender, HCP, diagnoses
Client's current baseline measurements, treatment plan, goals, and response to treatment
Priority and outstanding tasks and changes from previous days

Repositioning and transferring assigned patient by UAP's
RN must provide detailed instructions like when to move, which techniques to be used, and when to use assistive devices or persons.
Unstable clients and spinal cord stabilization (cervical collar) require the presence of the RN for repositioning or moving.
Guidelines to reduce risk of staff and client injury:
Use a gait/transfer belt to transfer a partially weight bearing client to a chair.
Use two or more caregivers to reposition clients who are uncooperative or unable to assist (sedated, comatose)
Use a full-body sling life to move/transfer nonparticipating clients.
Use two to three caregivers to move cooperative clients weighing less than 200 lbs.
Use three or more caregivers to move cooperative clients weighing more than 200 lbs.

Bishop score for induction of labor
The bishop score is a system for the assessment and rating of cervical favorability and readiness for induction of labor. The cervix is scored (0–3) on consistency, position, dilation, effacement, and station of the fetal presenting part. A higher Bishop score indicates an increase likelihood of successful induction that result in vaginal birth. For nulliparous women, a score greater than or equal to eight usually indicates that induction will be successful.
Note: A cervix that is firm and posterior is associated with a low Bishop score, which reflects low likelihood of successful labor induction

Cervix	Bishop score			
	0	1	2	3
Consistency	Firm	Medium	Soft	—
Position	Posterior	Mid-position	Anterior	—
Dilation	0 cm	1-2 cm	3-4 cm	≥5 cm
Effacement	0%-30%	40%-50%	60%-70%	≥80%
Station	−3	−2	−1, 0	+1, +2

Assessment and rating of cervical favorability and readiness for induction of labor
A higher bishop score indicates an increased likelihood of successful induction that results in vaginal birth.
For nulliparous women, a score greater than eight indicates that induction will be successful.

Opioid medications (Mo So4 etc.)

Nausea and vomiting are expected side effects when initiated treatment; however tolerance develops and persistent nausea is rare.
Take with an antiemetic and not in an empty stomach.
N/V are decreased when the client lies still in a flat position.

Physical assessment of a toddler

The order of examination is from least to most invasive.
Have the parents remove the clothing.
Allow the child to touch new pieces of equipment while being used.
Parent involvement reduces anxiety and encourages cooperation.

Suicidal ideation

"There is no reason for me to go on" statement and giving away possessions.
Perform a suicidal risk assessment to ensure client safety.
RN can ask direct questions like "Do you feel like hurting yourself?" or "Do you have a plan to kill yourself?"
If the client has suicide plans, the RN needs to ask about the details.
The risk of a client completing suicide increases when the client has planned for a specific time and place, chosen a highly lethal method, chooses circumstances in which there would be little or no chance of interruption.

Chronic anxiety

Resilient people readily deal with the stress they face by using interventions such as DBE, meditation, thought interruption, and muscle relaxation.

Parkland formula for fluid resuscitation

The Parkland formula calculates the amount of fluid that should be administered to critically burned patients over the first twenty-four hours post-injury.

The Parkland formula is as follows: total crystalloid fluid (i.e., a solution with small molecules that can move into cells) over the first 24 hours = 4 milliliters x % TBSA (total body surface area burned) x body weight (kg). In children, the formula is edited to 3 ml x % TBSA x weight (kg). In most cases, lactated ringers (i.e., sodium chloride, sodium lactate, potassium chloride, and calcium chloride) are used. Hypoglycemia and electrolyte abnormalities can also be prevented in children by administering maintenance fluids composed of normal saline and 5 percent dextrose.

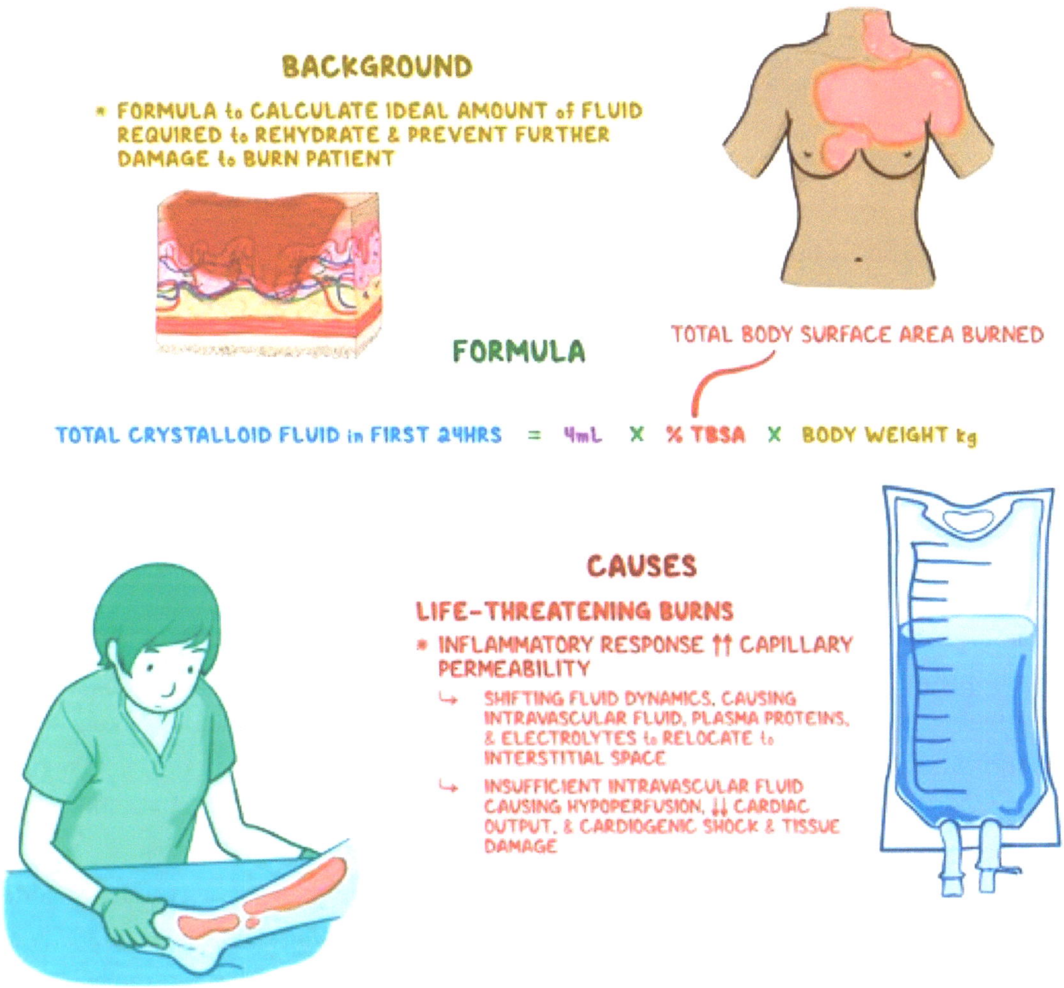

Schizophrenia affects a person's ability to think, speak, socialize, feel emotions, and perceive reality clearly. Schizophrenia patients may experience hallucinations, delusions, disorganized thinking, and difficulty concentrating. In addition to having trouble managing their behavior, they may also have difficulty deciding what to do. Neurotransmitter defects are also present in schizophrenia.**Schizophrenia is assessed by four A'S, each with many symptoms. The system of schizophrenia differs from person to person.**

Affect
Associative looseness
Autism
MBIVlence

A positive symptom is one that occurs when the disease is acutely onset, normal social function occurs during recovery, and the medication is well tolerated. Hallucination

Delusions
Illusion
Bizarre behavior

A negative symptom is one that occurs gradually over time, shows abnormal physical features, and responds poorly to treatments.

Apathy
Lack of motivation
Anhedonia
Poor thought process

Cognitive symptoms are common among schizophrenia patients. The issues they face include attention deficit disorder, memory loss, decision-making difficulties, and inability to solve issues.

Speech disorganization, disruptive behavior, and inappropriate affect are common symptoms of disorganization

Illusion As defined by general agreement, an illusion is a misrepresentation of a "real" sensory stimulus. Children may have illusions when they perceive tree branches at night as goblins. Imagination and cognitive processes in young minds result in these illusions as a normal part of childhood development.

Hallucination is a false perception which the person believes is real. Examples include seeing things, hearing things, feeling, tasteing, and smelling thing that are not there, i.e., a woman carried on a conversation with "her voices" while sitting alone in the hall.

Hallucination is a perception that is false, but that the person believes to be true. It is possible to see, hear, feel, taste, and smell things that are not there, e.g., a woman talked to herself in the hall while sitting alone.

Delusion: The term delusion refers to a false belief that an individual holds regardless of any reality testing that might challenge it. No social group supports the belief, regardless of evidence or arguments against it. It may reduce anxiety as it gives the individual the feeling of control, i.e., a man believes that he is Jesus and has been sent by God to help mankind. He spends hours reading his Bible and avoiding people.

Loose associations: In loose associations, there seems to be little connection between the thoughts, and it seems as though they are unrelated or have strange, unusual or illogical meanings. I.e. "I am in pain, Kams Jackson ... my migraine headache is on sumatriptan and off to the circus we wiggle."

Neologism: A private understanding of the meaning of a word that has been made up or vented by the individual. Example "spoon + fork = spork; I hate all the nurkeys on the unit." A concrete thinking approach relies on specific details to answer a question rather than abstracting the thought. An example of schizophrenia is the concrete thinking approach. People with schizophrenia have difficulty understanding abstract ideas and often have difficulty with reasoning. They also tend to have difficulty problem solving and making decisions and may be overwhelmed by small details. Example when asked by the physician how he was feeling, the man began to rub his arm and then answer "okay, soft I guess."

Echolalia - the repetition of whatever is said to them.

Word salad: A mixture of words that are totally without meaning for both the individual and listener; gibberish

Affect: Emotional feeling and gestures Mood: attitude and outlook on life.
In schizophrenia, ambivalence occurs when two opposing feelings are experienced at once. As an example, a patient gives the nurse 48 hours' notice
that he/she intends to leave. He then tells the nurse he has moved her bed closer to the window for a better view.
Waxy Flexibility: when a patient is catatonic, one can position a body part and the patient will hold it indefinitely. Clang Association: words used all rhyming_ soon, coon, goon, moon Depersonalization: person experiences body as being strange, unfamiliar, or as changing Derealization: Person does not feel real, feels like an actor on stage, or like he's living in a dream. Command Hallucinations: Voices that direct the individual to act. Threats by voices if demands are not met (suicidal/homicidal)

Strategy for answering Psychiatric questions.
Nursing Intervention for patient with Hallucinating

Look for clues like murmuring to oneself, looking around the room, tilting the head, or withdrawing behavior that indicates exhaustion.

Pay attention to the events that trigger hallucinations: isolation, stress, anger, and loss.

Ask directly if the person is experiencing hallucinations, e.g., "Are you hearing voices?"? Can you tell me what they are saying to you?"

Do not react to their voices as if they were real. Do not dispute their views. Refer to them as not real.

Respect the patient's feelings but express your own perspective: "You look very scared and worried, but there is no one else in this room." I feel safe in this place.

Make sure you are focusing on topics with real-world applications. I would like you to listen to my voice now. I need to talk to you."

Focus on the present moment by listening to music, counting backwards from 100, reading aloud, and singing.

Nursing Interventions for patient with Delusions

- To reduce suspiciousness, be open, honest, and reliable in interactions.
- Respond in a matter-of-fact way to suspicions.
- Avoid arguing about content of delusion.
- Focus on feelings. State, "It must be very frightening to think people are out to get you. I will not hurt you."
- Once the patient has described a delusion, do not dwell on it. Focus on reality-based subjects. If the client is obsessing with delusion, set limits on the amount of time devoted to delusion.
- Observe events that trigger delusions.
- Validate reality – "Yes, there was a funny smell in the dining. It was from the exterminator spraying for bugs."
- The activities you can engage with a patient that help to reduce delusional thoughts.:
- Computer games
- Chess
- Math problems
- Exercise
- Relaxation techniques

THREE TYPES OF SCHIZOPHRENIA

- Paranoid Schizophrenic

Catatonic Schizophrenia

Disorganized schizophrenia

Nursing Process with the paranoid schizophrenic patient

Thoughts:

- Hallucinations
- Delusions:
- Ideals of reference
- Thought broadcasting.
- Behavior:
- Poor eye contact
- Violence or suicidal
- Activities of daily leaving, self-directed
- Nursing Diagnosis
- Potential for violence, self-directed or at others related to:
- Command hallucination.
- Delusional thinking
- Lack of trust
- Panic anxiety.
- Altered thought process related to perceptual and cognitive distortions.

Nursing Interventions / Implementations

Provide safe environment:

- Quite room / low stimulation
- Monitor patient frequently.
- Remove all sharp objects from the room
- Redirect energy to physical outlet
- Non-competitive games
- Encourage exercise program to keep them busy
- Give the patient medication.
- Provide quit room
- Place them in isolation
- Restraints may be used
- Keep group activities to a minimum

- Give the patient mentally challenging activities
- Computer games, puzzles, and math problems
- Use honesty and consistent approach.
- Maintain a positive attitude throughout the process
- Avoid warm and fulsome statements
- You must not touch each other
- Maintain boundaries between your ego and others
- Ensure adequate space is available between you and the patient.
- Limit patient choices as much as possible
- Ensure their safety by taking the least restrictive measures possible
- It is important to consider the patient's feelings rather than the delusion.
- Your communication with the patient should be clear, simple, and straightforward.

When responding to infuriating or offensive verbal attacks, don't defend yourself

Evaluation/Outcome

- The patient will maintain control over his or her aggressive behavior to prevent harm to himself or others
- The patient's delusions will not interfere with their ability to perform daily tasks.

NEXT GENERATION NCLEX CASE STUDY
CRITICAL THINKING CASE STUDY

The **NEXT GENERATION NCLEX** is a comprehensive online course that provides nursing students with the knowledge and skills needed to pass the NCLEX-RN exam. It includes case studies, practice tests, tips and strategies to help students prepare for the exam. The course is designed to help students understand the content and setting of the NCLEX-RN exam. It also helps students build critical thinking and clinical judgment skills necessary to pass the exam. Additionally, the course provides students with guidance on test taking strategies to maximize their performance. Students who complete the course will be better prepared and more confident when taking the NCLEX-RN exam. They will be able to identify their strengths and weaknesses and develop an individualized plan for success.

CLINICAL JUDGEMENT is the observed outcome of critical thinking and decision making. It is an interactive process that uses nursing knowledge to observe and assess presenting situations.

It also generates the best evidence-based solutions to deliver safe client care. Improvements will be achieved through case studies, simulations, and other hands-on activities. Students will gain a deeper understanding of the concepts covered and be better able to apply them to real-life situations.

It is essential that students can practice their clinical judgement and hone their decision-making skills. This will help ensure that they are well equipped to handle any situation that may arise in their future professional practice.
The focus is critical thinking and decision-making ability.

What are the six NCSBN Clinical Judgement?
Measurement Model Cognitive Skill.

Recognize cues, i.e., ability to analyze
Analyze cues
Prioritize hypotheses
Generate solutions
Take action (nursing interventions)
Evaluate outcomes

Next Generation NCLEX TIPS 1
Recognize Cues

Remember to recognize cues, carefully review the client's assessment data like developmental age and history to help determine if findings are relevant or of immediate concern to the nurse. The NSCBN will give you a lot of information and only about 3 percent of the information is relevant and the rest of it is not important.

Analyze Cues

The nurse organizes and links them to the clients presenting clinical situation. Ask yourself: what does that relevant client data mean or indicate currently? Remember the NCLEX test nursing diagnoses and nursing interventions. Not medical diagnosis but sometimes the NCLEX can include some difficult question that has medical diagnosis like:

Client findings	Dehydration	Hypernatremia	Anemia
General weakness	✓	✓	✓
Acute Confusion	✓	✓	✓
Dry mouth	✓	✓	✓
Increase Heart rate	✓	✓	✓
Dyspnea on exertion			✓

The question may be asked on how the clinical manifestation of those symptoms related to other medical conditions. In the above items listed on the table, you used to ask yourself where I see…
Generalized weakness on dehydration, hyperthermia, or anemia
Acute condition
Prioritize hypotheses: The next cognitive skill requires you to narrow down what the data and priority the client's problems or needs.
Example:
A thirty-six-year-old postpartum client who just gave birth to a third child in five years report. Severe "after birth pain" of 9/10 on a 0 to 10 pain intensity scale. The client also reports having problems with getting the baby to latch for breast feeding/chest feeding. The nurse assesses that the client has a boggy uterus and is saturating a peri-pad every twenty to thirty minutes.

Prioritize – what is going on with the client?
Choose your key words from the scenarios.
Use Maslow's hierarchy of needs
First : saturating, bleeding
Second, severe pain
Third, teaching the client the proper technique of breastfeeding

Generate Solutions
After identifying the client's priority problem in a given clinical scenario, you want to think about all the possible actions that can be used to resolve or manage the problem (nursing intervention).

NEXT GENERATION NCLEX TIP 2

Remember to generate solutions to meet a client's priority need; determine the client's desired or expected outcomes first.

Take Action:

Deciding which action to implement is the focus of this clinical judgement thinking skill. After generating a list of possible interventions determine the most appropriate intervention or combination of interventions that will resolve or manage the client's priority health problems or concerns.

NEXT GENERATION NCLEX TIP 3

Remember: When deciding to take action, avoid memorized textbook methods and procedures. Instead, customize your action to meet the needs of the client in the clinical scenario.

EVALUATE OUTCOMES

The last clinical judgement thinking skill is to determine if the interventions implemented for the client resolved or effectively managed the health problems. The best way to make the determination is to compare what make the desired or expected outcomes are with current client findings or observed outcomes.

Ask yourself, "Which assessment findings/signs and symptoms indicate that the client's condition has improved? Which findings indicate that the client's condition has declined?"

How will the six clinical judgement skill be measured on the NGN?

NGN will measure clinical judgement through use of a variety of new test item types that are embedded into two types of case studies.

The unfolding case studies

The stand-alone items

Both types of cases present a clinical scenario and include part of a medical record like the record shows in the figure, e.g. health history, nurses notes, vital signs, laboratory results.

CASE STUDY

There are two types of case studies used on the NGN:

The stand-alone items

The unfolding case studies

Although there are some differences between the two types of cases, both types present a realistic clinical situation commonly encountered in practice by the new nursing graduate.

DIFFERENT BETWEEN STAND-ALONE ITEMS AND UNFOLDING CASE STUDIES

The unfolding case study presents the client situation over time through several phases of care in the clinical scenario (referred to as the NGN case study).

The client may initially be evaluated in an ED, in an acute care hospital, in a clinic, at school, in an urgent care center, or at home. As the scenario changes, or "unfolds," NGN test items required you to use all of the information including the information in the current phase of the clients care to answer each question.

Remember to first identify normal/usual or abnormal and expected (not relevant) and abnormal and not expected (relevant) client findings requiring follow-up.

Note the strategy words that indicate a complication (severe vs. mild/history of vs. now reports, etc.).

Pay attention to information provided in other tabs, nurse's notes, doctor's orders, tab reports, etc.

CASE STUDY

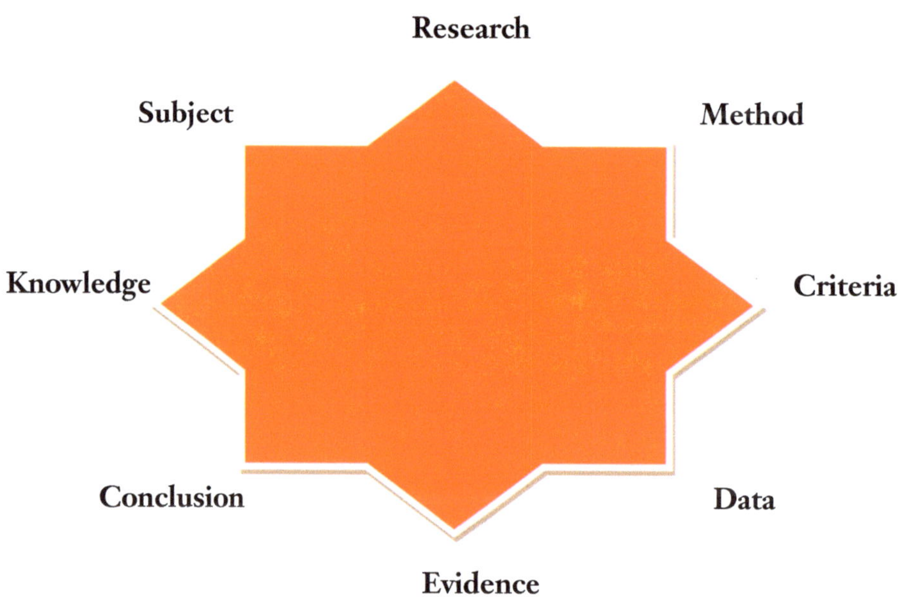

Note: The unfolding case study looks alike.

Mr. Britton Mike, a seventy-year-old white man has a history of mitral value regurgitation and left ventricular failure. Mr. Britton came to the emergency dept (ED) with symptoms of increasing shortness of breath over the past week and was transferred to the ICU. The ICU nurse immediately goes to check on Mr. Britton and noticed the following:

He indicated that he feels very short of breath.

He was lying in bed, pale with circumoral cyanosis, and respirations appeared labored and rapid.

ER nurses notes:

The client is awake and alert.

Vital signs taken: BP 110/85, HR 110 O2 Stat 89, RR 26, Furosemide 100 mg IV administered, oxygen via nasal cannula administered at 4 L/min.

Explanation:
First do the key words:
What action should the ICU nurse take first: priority?
Listen to the breath sounds.
Ask when the dyspnea started.
Check the oxygen saturation.
Place the check in high fowlers position. Correct (ABC)
This is a priority question, you can use:
Assessment vs Implementation, ABC, Maslow Hierarchy of need or SAARED methods strategy
Two hours later, the nurse reassesses Mr. Mike Britton and notices the following:
Crackles audible throughout both lung fields.
Client is coughing up pink frothy sputum.
Jugular vein distention
BP 115/85; HR 108/min
Peripheral pulse 2/4 with a capillary refill time < 3 seconds
Oxygen saturation is 85% with the oxygen at 4 L/min per the nasal cannula
Respiratory rate is 38 breaths/min.
3 + to 4 + pitting edema in her feet and up to midcalf

Based on Mr. Mike's history and assessment, the nurse will be most concerned about which complication?
Pulmonary edema Correct
Cardiac Tamponade
Pneumonia
Pulmonary embolus

Based on client's current medical condition, which action will the nurse take next?
Activate the hospital's Rapid Response Team (RRT).
Switch to a nonrebreather mass at an O_2 flow rate OF 15 L/min.
Assist the client to cough and deep breathe.
Administer the prescribed morphine sulfate 2 mg IV to the client.

Rationale:
Think of something that you can do now that will help the client. Use the elimination process to choose the correct option. Option 2 is the correct answer. This indicates that the priority here is to give the client a higher O_2 using nonrebreather mass.

Fifteen minutes after, the client's condition is the following:

Patient is confused.
Labor Led Respirations
BP 81/41 HR 65 RR 33 O2 SAT. 85
ABGs PH 7.31 PCO2 60 HCO3 24 PAO2 64
Creatinine 1.1 mg/mL
Na+: 133 mEq /L K+: 5.2 mEq/L

The doctor places new orders:

Repeat administration of furosemide 100 mg IV
Insert a 16 French urinary Foley Catheter
12 lead ECG
Help patients with endotracheal intubation. Correct
Bolus administration of ringer Lactate with albumin 5 percent.
Rational: Highlight which doctors order will the nurse implement first? This patient needs intubation.

The nurse comes back that day for another shift and is taking care of Mr. Mike again.
The nurse assesses the following: Which data indicates improvement or no improvement?

Upon morning rounds the HCP has determined to transfer Mr. Mike to the step-down cardiac unit for several days prior to being discharged.

Prior to transferring Mr. Mike to the step-down unit, the nurse should take which of the following actions? **Select all that apply.**
Take the clients vital signs. Correct
Notify the client's family of the transfer. Correct
Call the step-down unit's nurse and give nurse the report. Correct
Remove cardiac telemetry monitor prior to the transfer.
Request the UAP to gather the client's personal items to be transferred with the client. Correct

HOW DO YOU KNOW WHEN TO PRIORITIZE:

In the NCLEX the examiner will give you a question. For instance:

Key words you need to know when to prioritize:

Which patient will you see or assess first?

Which patient will have the highest priority?

Which patient will you administer medication first?

You are given an assignment for the nursing shift. You are expected to prioritize clients' needs. These needs are for a group of clients and determine which assigned client you will need to **ASSESS OR SEE FIRST?**

Client being discharged to home today who needs further teaching about insulin administration and diet.

Client who was admitted to the nursing unit during evening because of difficult breathing. CORRECT

Client on IV antibiotics and due to receive a dose at 0900.

First highlight the key words and use the elimination method and choose the correct option.

How to Analyze Cues

Analyzing the cues in a question allows you to identify what is relevant or not relevant in the question. Also, this process determines what relevant data means and tells you what is happening to the customer. Once this is determined, you can determine what you need to plan and do next to meet the client's needs. The analysis of cues can also help to identify potential problems that the client may be experiencing. This can help to address the problem faster and more effectively. Finally, it can provide insight into potential solutions that may be suitable for the client.

Question 1.

A forty-two-year-old client is admitted to the acute behavioral health unit for observation and therapy. The client is accompanied by their sibling, who tells the nurse that the client has had a noticeable in-characteristic change in behavior over the last four to five days. The nurse cares for the client during the daytime shift and provides the oncoming nurse with a report on the client.

Nurses note: Client was talking and cracking jokes with everyone, demand another client's attention. Making inappropriate sexual propositions to the other clients sitting in the day room. Telling everyone they are the child of the vice president of the United States. Too distracted and disorganized to eat lunch. Writing numerous letters to famous people in Hollywood. Overactive and busily occupied with grandiose plans. Verbalizing crude and sexual remarks and profanities to the nursing staff.

For each assessment finding, click to specify if the finding is consistent with hypomania or acute mania.

NEXT GENERATION NCLEX CASE STUDY QUESTIONS

Case study | Question 1 - Choose the most appropriate response.

As a nurse, you are completing your nursing actions, and you hear the ventilator alarm sound. You identify it as a high pressure alarm.

What is your first step?

1. Call the doctor.

2. Assess the patient. Correct

3. Administer oxygen.

4. Turn the alarm off.

Rational: Conducting a thorough assessment of the patient will help determine the cause of the high pressure alarm. The patient's vital signs should be monitored and checked for any abnormalities. Any changes in the patient's condition should be reported to a doctor immediately. If the patient requires further treatment, they should be transported to an emergency room.

Case study | Question 2 - Choose the most appropriate response.

In the process of assessing your patient, you note that gauze obstructs the view of the trach stoma. The ventilator alarms "High Pressure" continuously.

What is the next appropriate course of action?

Check the patient's vitals.

Verify the trach is connected correctly. Correct

Try to silence and turn off the ventilator alarm to ensure it works properly.

Ask the caregiver if this happens often.

Rational: It is critical to always start by assessing your patient's airway first. You should check the trach to verify placement and ensure the ventilator is properly connected. If necessary, remove any object that may obstruct the view of the trach being inserted into the stoma. This includes gauze, clothing, blankets, etc.

Case Study | Question 3 - Choose the most appropriate response.

During this assessment of the patient's breath sounds, you noted rhonchi throughout. Now that you have identified the potential cause of the high pressure alarm, you can take the appropriate actions to resolve the situation.
What should your next step be?

Reposition the patient.

Administer PRN bronchodilators.

Call the physician.

Suction the trach. Correct

Rational: By suctioning the trach, you clear the airway, improve airflow, and decrease pressure. You have now successfully resolved the cause of this high pressure alarm.

Case Study | Question 4 - Choose the most appropriate response.

After verifying your patient's trach placement and assessing breath sounds, you note clear, but diminished breath sounds throughout. The patient's chest rise is regular and symmetrical. The low pressure alarm sounds continuously.
What is your next step?

Suction the trach.

Assess the circuit connections. Correct

Drain any excess water from the ventilator circuit.

Call the caregiver for assistance.

Rational: Starting at the trach and working toward the vent, check all the circuit connections and accessories. By tightening the loose connections, you resolved the low pressure alarm. By beginning your investigation at the patient and continuing from there, you have successfully found the cause of the low pressure alarm. Working your way through the different potential causes prevents a situation from becoming worse.

Case Study | Question 5 - Choose the most appropriate response.

You complete the repositioning of your patient, and you notice that the ventilator starts alarming "low pressure." **What is your first step to resolve this issue?**

Change the trach.

Assess the patient. Correct

Assess the ventilator tubing for disconnection.

Silence and reset the alarm.

Rational: It is imperative to verify that the trach is properly placed and connected to the vent circuit.

Case Study | Question 6- Choose the most appropriate response.

You notice a diminished breath sound and shallow respirations upon assessing the patient. Based on these findings, you remove the split gauze from the trach. You observe that the trach has dislodged from the stoma but is still connected to the ventilator. **What is your next course of action?**

Apply Oxygen via blow-by.

Assess the patient's additional vital signs.

Immediately reinsert the trach.

Disconnect the vent tubing and insert the backup trach with an obturator. Correct

Rational: Inserting the same-sized trach with an obturator is the most recommended practice. It may be necessary to reinsert the dislodged trach with an obturator if a backup trach is unavailable. It is imperative to save the obturator and always keep it with the patient as part of their essential trach equipment for reinsertion.

Case Study | Question 7- Choose the most appropriate response.

You have a backup trach of the same size ready to be used. You oxygenate the patient prior to changing the trach. But, once you remove the trach, you find it difficult to reinsert the trach of the same size. A one-size-smaller emergency trach is inserted, although with some difficulty. The patient's stomachs are now inflamed and bleeding from the site. As you are almost finished securing the trach ties, the patient coughs it out. The pulse oximeter is alarming with oxygen saturation dropping below 85%. The heart rate which was previously tachycardic is now bradycardic and the heart rate is now 50 BPM. The patient has lost consciousness and has become cyanotic. The patient's family is frantic, screaming, and crying at this point. Time is running out, and you have a limited window to act. **What should your next action be?**

Cover the stoma site with your gloved finger and ventilate the patient using the ambu bag with face mask and max oxygen meter flow while the other nurse calls 911 EMS.

Start bagging the stoma site with maximum oxygen meter flow ordered via the ambu bag. Tell the nurse to call 911 EMS.

Cover the stoma with gloved fingers, start CPR (while providing breathing only), tell the other nurse to call 911 EMS, and then have her assist with bagging the client using the face mask attached to the ambu bag and oxygen per order. Correct

Rational: In all alarm scenarios, you always start with the patient. In this case, it is incredibly imperative to also perform CPR, based on the patient's age and their heart rate being less than 60 BPM. It is important to assess the patient's breathing and circulation before performing CPR. It is also important to make sure that the patient's airway is clear before administering rescue breaths. Finally, it is important to monitor the patient's vital signs until help arrives.

The Future of Nursing 2020–2030: Charting a Path to Achieve Health Equity.
Nursing's capacity and expertise will help it contribute meaningfully to health equity, according to the Committee on the Future of Nursing 2020–2030 (The National Academy of Science, Engineering and Medicine, 2021). This report provides recommendations to improve nurses' diversity, education, and collaboration to better meet the evolving needs of the healthcare system. It focuses on how nurses can contribute to health equity and reduce care disparities. It further highlights the importance of adequate staffing and training in nursing. It emphasizes the need for nurses to be aware of and sensitive to cultural and linguistic differences to provide equitable care. Nurses should also be given the resources they need to stay up to date on the latest advances in nursing care. Lastly, nurses should be empowered to advocate for their patients and their profession. All these factors contribute to an environment that promotes quality patient care. Nurses should also be supported in their efforts to practice evidence-based care, which can lead to improved healthcare outcomes. Furthermore, nurses should be encouraged to pursue professional development opportunities to further their knowledge and skills. Nurses should be provided with the resources and support necessary to ensure they can provide quality care to their patients. They should also be given the freedom to make patient care decisions. Finally, they should be celebrated and recognized for their work and dedication (The National Academy of Science, Engineering and Medicine, 2021).

The trend occurring in the nursing workforce and how nursing education is adapting to meet the evolving needs of the profession.

Nursing education is evolving to include more technology-driven and evidence-based practices. Nurses are also being encouraged to take a more active role in leading change by advocating for patients and engaging in research. Nurses are uniquely positioned to provide insight and guidance on the changing healthcare landscape. Nurses are expected to be lifelong learners, adapting to the changing needs of their patients and the healthcare system. They are also expected to be leaders in their profession, leading the way in implementing new technologies and evidence-based practices. This speaks to the importance of nursing education in preparing nurses for the future of healthcare.

A growing number of women and members of historically underrepresented groups are working in the field of nursing. Due to these factors, nursing schools now offer degree programs that are designed for working people, with flexible scheduling and online learning options available. Women and people of color have played a significant role in nursing's development. Increasing numbers of women of color are entering the nursing profession, which is expected to continue. As a result, minority populations are predicted to rise in the coming years, following American demographic trends (American Association of Colleges of Nursing, 2023). This will help to enhance cultural competence in the nursing profession, which is essential for providing quality healthcare to diverse communities. Diversity in the nursing profession will also help to address healthcare disparities faced by minority and underserved populations. It can also increase diverse voices representation in the healthcare industry (American Association of Colleges of Nursing, 2023).

As students' work schedules and family obligations have evolved, nursing schools have supplied them with more flexibility. Students with busy schedules and working professionals can also benefit from hybrid and online nursing courses offered by nursing schools. There are an increasing number of nursing programs available for working adults who want to switch careers or go back to school after an extended absence. To meet the demand for a more diverse nursing workforce, nursing schools enable a wider range of people to enter the profession. The nursing profession is becoming increasingly diverse, and nurses need to encourage their colleagues to embrace diversity and inclusion. Further, nurses play an essential role in advancing evidence-based practice, which leads to an improved outcome for patients. In addition, nurses need to be aware of how cultural biases can affect patient care and be open to learning about different cultures and beliefs. They should also strive to create a safe and comfortable environment for all patients and colleagues by embracing diversity and inclusion (American Association of Colleges of Nursing, 2023).

Moreover, nurses may serve as mentors and role models for other health care workers. Keeping up with the latest developments in their field is an essential part of being an effective change agent. It is equally important that they communicate their vision for the future of the profession. As part of the healthcare team, nurses must be willing to collaborate and share ideas (The National Academy of Science, Engineering and Medicine, 2021). Nurses can help the healthcare system adapt to the constantly changing demands of the healthcare profession by supporting its requirements, promoting evidence-based practice, and recruiting skilled nurses. Nurses should also encourage the use of technology to improve patient care and outcomes, while continuing to provide the vital human touch that only a nurse can. They should strive to stay informed and be willing to take risks to bring about positive changes (The National Academy of Science, Engineering and Medicine, 2021).

JACKS NCLEX REVIEW

EXAM: NCLEX

TITLE: RN/PN PRACTICE EXAM

1) A male client is admitted to the psychiatric unit after experiencing severe depression. He states that he intends to kill himself, but he asks the nurse not to repeat his intentions to other staff members. Which response demonstrates understanding and appropriate action on the part of the nurse?
A. "I understand you're depressed but killing yourself is not a reasonable option."
B. "We need to discuss this further, but right now let's complete these forms."
C. "Don't do that, you have so much to live for. You have a wonderful wife and children. The client in the next room has no one."
D. "This is very serious. I do not want any harm to come to you. I will have to report this to the rest of the staff."

2) A depressed client is seen at the mental health center for follow-up after an attempted suicide one week ago. She has taken phenelzine sulfate (Nardil), a monoamine oxidase (MAO) inhibitor, for seven straight days. She states that she is not feeling any better. The nurse explains that the drug must accumulate to an effective level before symptoms are totally relieved. Symptom relief is expected to occur within:
10 days
2-4 weeks
2 months
3 months

3) Cystic fibrosis is transmitted as an autosomal recessive trait. This means that:
A. Mothers carry the gene and pass it to their sons.
B. Fathers carry the gene and pass it to their daughters.
C. Both parents must have the disease for a child to have the disease.
D. Both parents must be carriers for a child to have the disease.

4) A twenty-four-year-old client presents to the emergency department protesting, "I am God."The nurse identifies this as a:
A. Delusion
B. Illusion
C. Hallucination
D. Conversion

5) In acute episodes of mania, lithium is effective in one to two weeks, but it may take up to four weeks, or even a few months, to treat symptoms fully. Sometimes an antipsychotic agent is prescribed during the first few days or weeks of an acute episode to manage severe behavioral excitement and acute psychotic symptoms. In addition to the lithium, which one of the following medications might the physician prescribe?

A. Diazepam (Valium)
B. Haloperidol (Haldol)
C. Sertraline (Zoloft)
D. Alprazolam (Xanax)

6) A violent client remains in restraints for several hours. Which of the following interventions is most appropriate while he is in restraints?
A. Give fluids if the client requests them.
B. Assess skin integrity and circulation of extremities before applying restraints and as they are removed.
C. Measure vital signs at least every four hours.
D. Release restraints every two hours for client to exercise.

7) The pediatrician has diagnosed tinea capitis in an eight-year-old girl and has placed her on oral griseofulvin. The nurse should emphasize which of these instructions to the mother and/or child?
A. Administer oral griseofulvin on an empty stomach for best results.
B. Discontinue drug therapy if food tastes funny.
C. May discontinue medication when the child experiences symptomatic relief.
D. Observe for headaches, dizziness, and anorexia.

8) A client with cirrhosis of the liver becomes comatose and is started on neomycin 300 mg q6h via nasogastric tube. The rationale for this therapy is to:
A. Prevent systemic infection
B. Promote diuresis
C. Decrease ammonia formation
D. Acidify the small bowel

9) A five-year-old has just had a tonsillectomy and adenoidectomy. Which of these nursing measures should be included in postoperative care?
A. Encourage the child to cough up blood if present.
B. Give warm clear liquids when fully alert.
C. Have the child gargle and do toothbrushing to remove old blood.
D. Observe for evidence of bleeding.

10) A sixteen-month-old infant is being prepared for tetralogy of Fallot repair. In the nursing assessment, which lab value should elicit further assessment and requires notification of physician?
A. pH 7.39
B. White blood cell (WBC) count 10,000 WBCs/mm3
C. Hematocrit 60%

D. Bleeding time of 4 minutes

11) A male client is experiencing extreme distress. He begins to pace up and down the corridor. What nursing intervention is appropriate when communicating with a pacing client?
A. Ask him to sit down. Speak slowly and use short, simple sentences.
B. Help him to recognize his anxiety.
C. Walk with him as he paces.
D. Increase the level of his supervision.

12) Prior to an amniocentesis, a fetal ultrasound is done to:
A. Evaluate fetal lung maturity.
B. Evaluate the amount of amniotic fluid.
C. Locate the position of the placenta and fetus.
D. Ensure that the fetus is mature enough to perform the amniocentesis.

13) A twenty-five-year-old client believes she may be pregnant with her first child. She schedules an obstetric examination with the nurse practitioner to determine the status of her possible pregnancy. Her last menstrual period began May 20, and her estimated date of confinement using Nagele's rule is:
A. March 27
B. February 1
C. February 27
D. January 3

14) A client is now pregnant for the second time. Her first child weighed 4536 g. at delivery. The client's glucose tolerance test shows elevated blood sugar levels. Because she only shows signs of diabetes when she is pregnant, she is classified as having:
A. Insulin-dependent diabetes
B. Type II diabetes mellitus
C. Type I diabetes mellitus
D. Gestational diabetes mellitus

15) A forty-four-year-old female client is receiving external radiation to her scapula for metastasis of breast cancer. Teaching related to skin care for the client would include which of the following?
A. Teach her to completely clean the skin to remove all ointments and markings after each treatment.
B. Teach her to cover broken skin in the treated area with a medicated ointment.
C. Encourage her to wear a tight-fitting vest to support her scapula.
D. Encourage her to avoid direct sunlight on the area being treated.

16) The nurse is assisting a fourth-day postoperative cholecystectomy client in planning her meals for tomorrow's menu. Which vitamin is the most essential in promoting tissue healing?
Vitamin C
Vitamin B1
Vitamin D
Vitamin A

17) A ten-year-old client with a pin in the right femur is immobilized in traction. He is exhibiting behavioral changes including restlessness, difficulty with problem solving, inability to concentrate on activities, and monotony. Which of the following nursing implementations would be most effective in helping him cope with immobility?
A. Providing him with books, challenging puzzles, and games as diversionary activities
B. Allowing him to do as much for himself as he is able, including learning to do pin-site care under supervision
C. Having a volunteer come in to sit with the client and to read him stories
D. Stimulating rest and relaxation by gentle rubbing with lotion and changing the client's position frequently

18) In client teaching, the nurse should emphasize that fetal damage occurs more frequently with ingestion of drugs during:
A. First trimester
B. Second trimester
C. Third trimester
D. Every trimester

19) On admission, the client has signs and symptoms of pulmonary edema. The nurse places the client in the most appropriate position for a client in pulmonary edema, which is:
A. High Fowler
B. Lying on the left side
C. Sitting in a chair
D. Supine with feet elevated

20) A client has returned to the unit from the recovery room after having a thyroidectomy. The nurse knows that a major complication after a thyroidectomy is:
A. Respiratory obstruction
B. Hypercalcemia
C. Fistula formation
D. Myxedema

21) The nurse should facilitate bonding during the postpartum period. What should the nurse expect to observe in the taking-hold phase?
A. Mother is concerned about her recovery.
B. Mother calls infant by name.
C. Mother lightly touches infant.
D. Mother is concerned about her weight gain.

22) A female client has just died. Her family is requesting that all nursing staff leave the room. The family's religious leader has arrived and is ready to conduct a ceremony for the deceased in the room, requesting that only family members be present. The nurse assigned to the client should perform the appropriate nursing action, which might include:
A. Inform the family that it is the hospital's policy not to conduct religious ceremonies in client rooms.
B. Refuse to leave the room because the client's body is entrusted in the nurse's care until it can be brought to the morgue.
C. Tell the family that they may conduct their ceremony in the client's room; however, the nurse must attend.
D. Respect the client's family's wishes.

23)A woman diagnosed with multiple sclerosis is disturbed with diplopia. The nurse will teach her to:
A. Limit activities that require focusing (close vision)
B. Take more frequent naps
C. Use artificial tears
D. Wear a patch over one eye

24) One of the most reliable assessment tools for adequacy of fluid resuscitation in burned children is:
A. Blood pressure
B. Level of consciousness
C. Skin turgor
D. Fluid intake

25) A client with a diagnosis of C-4 injury has been stabilized and is ready for discharge. Because this client is at risk for autonomic dysreflexia, he and his family should be instructed to assess for and report:
A. Dizziness and tachypnea
B. Circumoral pallor and lightheadedness
C. Headache and facial flushing
D. Pallor and itching of the face and neck.

Reference

Silvestri, Linda Anne. *Saunders Comprehensive Review for the NCLEX Examination, 7TH Edition*. Elsevier, 2017.

Kockrow, Christensen. *Foundations of Nursing, 6th Edition*. Mosby Elsevier, 2011.

Carol, Taylor, Lillis Carol, and Lynn Pamela. *Fundamentals of Nursing: The Art and Science of Person-Centered Nursing Care*. 2015.

"Mortality in the United States, 2020." *U.S. Department of Health and Human Services Centers for Disease Control and Prevention.* **https://www.cdc.gov/nchs/data/databriefs/db427.pdf**

U.S. Preventive Services Taskforce (2023). Retrieved **https://www.uspreventiveservicestaskforce.org/uspstf/**

"Aspirin Use to Prevent Cardiovascular Disease: Preventative Medicine.". *Healthy People 2030*. Retrieved from **https://health.gov/healthypeople/tools-action/browse-evidence-based-resources/aspirin-use-prevent-cardiovascular-disease-and-colorectal-cancer-preventive-medication/**

Mosby's PDQ for RN: Nursing Facts at Hand, Fourth Edition. Elsevier, 2017.

"The Future of Nursing 2020-2030. Charting a Path to Achieve Health Equity." *The National Academy of Science, Engineering and Medicine*. Washington, DC: The National Academies Press, 2021.

La Charity, Linda A., Candice K. Kumagai, and Barbara Bartz. *Prioritization, Delegation, and Assignment: Practice Exercises for the NCLEX Examination, 5th Edition*. Elsevier, 2021.

Susan Scott Ricci, Terri Kyle, Susan Carman, 2017. Maternity and Pediatric Nursing, Third Edition. Wolters Kluwer

APPENDIX

NCLEX RN QUESTION ANSWERS AND RATIONALE

1. Answer: D
Explanation:
(A) To the client, suicide may be a reasonable action and the only one he can cope with at this time. (B) This response indicates to the client that his intention to commit suicide is not important to the nurse currently. (C) The client is so depressed that he is not able to see the positive aspects of his life. At no time should the nurse discuss another client's problems in conversation. (D) This statement tells the client that the nurse recognizes his problem is of a serious nature and will take all steps necessary to help him.

2. Answer: D
Explanation:
(A) This answer is incorrect. It can take up to one month for the therapeutic effect of the medication. (B) This answer is correct. Because MAO inhibitors are slow to act, it takes 2–4 weeks before improvement of symptoms is noted. (C) This answer is incorrect. It can take up to one month for the therapeutic effect of the medication. (D) This answer is incorrect. Therapeutic effects of the medication are noted within one month of drug therapy.

3. Answer: D
Explanation:
(A) Cystic fibrosis is not an X-linked or sex-linked disease. (B) The only characteristic on the Y chromosome is the trait for hairy ears. (C) Both parents do not need to have the disease but must be carriers. (D) If a trait is recessive, two genes (one from each parent) are necessary to produce an affected child.

4. Answer: A
Explanation:
(A) Delusion is a false belief. (B) Illusion is the misrepresentation of a real, external sensory experience. (C) Hallucination is a false sensory perception involving any of the senses. (D) Conversion is the expression of intrapsychic conflict through sensory or motor manifestations.

5. Answer: B

Explanation:

(A) Diazepam is an antianxiety medication and is not designed to reduce psychotic symptoms. (B) Haloperidol is an antipsychotic medication and may be used until lithium takes effect. (C) Sertraline is an antidepressant and is used primarily to reduce symptoms of depression. (D) Alprazolam is an antianxiety medication and is not designed to reduce psychotic symptoms.

6. Answer: D

Explanation:

(A) Fluids (nourishment) should be offered at regular intervals whether the client requests (or refuses) them or not. (B) Skin integrity and circulation of the extremities should be checked regularly while the client is restrained, not only before restraints are applied and after they are removed. (C) Vital signs should be checked at least every two hours. If the client remains agitated in restraints, vital signs should be monitored even more closely, perhaps every one to two hours. (D) Restraints should be released every two hours for exercise, one extremity at a time, to maintain muscle tone, skin and joint integrity, and circulation.

7. Answer: D

Explanation:

(A) Giving the drug with or after meals may allay gastrointestinal discomfort. Giving the drug with a fatty meal (ice cream or milk) increases absorption rate. (B) Griseofulvin may alter taste sensations and thereby decrease the appetite. Monitoring of food intake is important, and inadequate nutrient intake should be reported to the physician. (C) The child may experience symptomatic relief after 48–96 hours of therapy. It is important to stress continuing the drug therapy to prevent relapse (usually about six weeks). (D) The incidence of side effects is low; however, headaches are common. Nausea, vomiting, diarrhea, and anorexia may occur. Dizziness, although uncommon, should be reported to the physician.

8. Answer: C

Explanation:

(A) Neomycin is an antibiotic, but this is not the rationale for administering it to a client in hepatic coma. (B) Diuretics and salt-free albumin are used to promote diuresis in clients with cirrhosis of the liver. (C) Neomycin destroys the bacteria in the intestines. It is the bacteria in the bowel that breaks down protein into ammonia. (D) Lactulose is administered to create an acid environment in the bowel. Ammonia leaves the blood and migrates to this acidic environment where it is trapped and excreted.

9. Answer: D

Explanation:

(A) The nurse should discourage the child from coughing, clearing the throat, or putting objects in his mouth. These may induce bleeding. (B) Cool, clear liquids may be given when a child is fully alert. Warm liquids may dislodge a blood clot. The nurse should avoid red- or brown-colored liquids to distinguish fresh or old blood from ingested liquid should the child vomit. (C) Gargles and vigorous toothbrushing could initiate bleeding. (D) Postoperative hemorrhage, though unusual, may occur. The nurse should observe for bleeding by looking directly into the throat and for vomiting of bright red blood, continuous swallowing, and changes in vital signs.

10. Answer: C

Explanation:

(A) Normal pH of arterial blood gases for an infant are 7.35–7.45. (B) Normal white blood cell count in an infant is 6,000–17,500 WBCs/mm3. (C) Normal hematocrit in infant is 28%–42%. A 60% hematocrit may indicate polycythemia, a common complication of cyanotic heart disease. (D) Normal bleeding time is 2–7 minutes.

11. Answer: C

Explanation:

(A) The nurse should not ask him to sit down. Pacing is the activity he has chosen to deal with his anxiety. The nurse dealing with this client should speak slowly and with short, simple sentences. (B) The client may already recognize the anxiety and is attempting to deal with it. (C) Walk with the client as he paces. This gives support while he uses anxiety-generated energy. (D) Increasing the level of supervision may be appropriate after he stops pacing. It would minimize self-injury and/or loss of control.

12. Answer: C

Explanation:

(A) Amniocentesis can be performed to assess lung maturity. Fetal ultrasound can be used for gestational dating, although it does not separately determine lung maturity. (B) Ultrasound can evaluate amniotic fluid volume, which may be used to determine congenital anomalies. (C) Amniocentesis involves removal of amniotic fluid for evaluation. The needle, inserted through the abdomen, is guided by ultrasound to avoid needle injuries, and the test evaluates the position of the placenta and the fetus. (D) Amniocentesis can be performed as early as the fifteenth to the seventeenth week of pregnancy.

13. Answer: C
Explanation:
(A) March 27 is a miscalculation. (B) February 1 is a miscalculation. (C) February 27 is the correct answer. To calculate the estimated date of confinement using Nagele's rule, subtract three months from the date that the last menstrual cycle began and then add seven days to the result. (D) January 3 is a miscalculation.

14. Answer: D
Explanation:
(A) Insulin-dependent diabetes mellitus, also known as type I diabetes, usually appears before the age of thirty years with an abrupt onset of symptoms requiring insulin for management. It is not related to onset during pregnancy. (B) Non-insulin-dependent diabetes (type II diabetes) usually appears in older adults. It has a slow onset and progression of symptoms. (C) This type of diabetes is the same as insulin-dependent diabetes. (D) Gestational diabetes mellitus has its onset of symptoms during pregnancy and usually disappears after delivery. These symptoms are usually mild and not life threatening, although they are associated with increased fetal morbidity and other fetal complications.

15. Answer: D
Explanation:
(A) The skin in a treatment area should be rinsed with water and patted dry. Markings should be left intact, and the skin should not be scrubbed. (B) Clients should avoid putting any creams or lotions on the treated area. This could interfere with treatment. (C) Radiation therapy clients should wear loose fitting clothes and avoid tight, irritating fabrics. (D) The area of skin being treated is sensitive to sunlight, and the client should take care to prevent sun damage by avoiding direct sunlight and covering the area when she is in the sun.

16. Answer: A
Explanation:
(A) Vitamin C (ascorbic acid) is essential in promoting wound healing and collagen formation. (B) Vitamin B1 (thiamine) maintains normal gastrointestinal (GI) functioning, oxidizes carbohydrates, and is essential for normal functioning of nervous tissue. (C) Vitamin D regulates absorption of calcium and phosphorus from the GI tract and helps prevent rickets. (D) Vitamin A is necessary for the formation and maintenance of skin and mucous membranes. It is also essential for normal growth and development of bones and teeth.

17. Answer: B
Explanation:
(A) These activities could be frustrating for the client if he is having difficulty with problem solving and concentration. (B) Selfcare is usually well received by the child, and it is one of the most useful interventions to help the child cope with immobility. (C) This may be helpful to the client if he has no visitors, but it does little to help him develop coping skills. (D) This will help to prevent skin irritation or breakdown related to immobility but will not help to prevent behavioral changes related to immobility.

18. Answer: A
Explanation:
(A) Organogenesis occurs in the first trimester. Fetus is most susceptible to malformation during this period. (B) Organogenesis has occurred by the second trimester. (C) Fetal development is complete by this time. (D) The dangerous period for fetal damage is the first trimester, not the entire pregnancy.

19. Answer: A
Explanation:
(A) High Fowler position decreases venous return to the heart and permits greater lung expansion so that oxygenation is maximized. (B) Lying on the left side may improve perfusion to the left lung but does not promote lung expansion. (C) Sitting in a chair will decrease venous return and promote maximal lung expansion. However, clients with pulmonary edema can deteriorate quickly and require intubation and mechanical ventilation. If a client is sitting in a chair when this deterioration happens, it will be difficult to intervene quickly. (D) The supine with feet elevated position increases venous return and will worsen pulmonary edema.

20. Answer: A
Explanation:
(A) Respiratory obstruction due to edema of the glottis, bilateral laryngeal nerve damage, or tracheal compression from hemorrhage is a major complication after a thyroidectomy. (B) Hypocalcemia accompanied by tetany from accidental removal of one or more parathyroid glands is a major complication, not hypercalcemia. (C) Fistula formation is not a major complication associated with a thyroidectomy. It is a major complication with a laryngectomy. (D) Myxedema is hypothyroidism that occurs in adults and is not a complication of a thyroidectomy. A thyroidectomy client tends to develop thyroid storm, which is excess production of thyroid hormone.

21. Answer: B
Explanation:
(A) This observation can be made during the taking-in phase when the mother's needs are more important. (B) This observation can be made during the taking-hold phase when the mother is actively involved with herself and the infant. (C, D) This observation can be made during the taking-in phase.

22. Answer: D
Explanation:
(A) It is rare that a hospital has a specific policy addressing this issue. If the statement is true, the nurse should show evidence of the policy to the family and suggest alternatives, such as the hospital chapel. (B) Refusal to leave the room demonstrates a lack of understanding related to the family's needs to grieve in their own manner. (C) The nurse should leave the room and allow the family privacy in their grief. (D) The family's wish to conduct a religious ceremony in the client's room is part of the grief process. The request is based on specific cultural and religious differences dictating social customs.

23. Answer: D
Explanation:
(A) Limiting activities requiring close vision will not alleviate the discomfort of double vision. (B) Frequent naps may be comforting, but they will not prevent double vision. (C) Artificial tears are necessary in the absence of a corneal reflex, but they have no effect on diplopia. (D) An eye patch over either eye will eliminate the effects of double vision during the time the eye patch is worn. An eye patch is safe for a person with an intact corneal reflex.

24. Answer: B
Explanation:
(A) Blood pressure can remain normotensive in a state of hypovolemia. (B) Capillary refill, alterations in sensorium, and urine output are the most reliable indicators for assessing hydration. (C) Skin turgor is not a reliable indicator for assessing hydration in a burn client. (D) Fluid intake does not indicate adequacy of fluid resuscitation in a burn client.

25. Answer: C
Explanation:
(A) Tachypnea is not a symptom. (B) Circumoral pallor is not a symptom. (C) Autonomic dysreflexia is an uninhibited and exaggerated reflex of the autonomic nervous system to stimulation, which results in vasoconstriction and elevated blood pressure. (D) Pallor and itching are not symptoms.

INSTRUCTOR'S ADVICE

The Night Before Your Exam

You should relax and get a good night's sleep. Avoid studying late into the night and get enough rest.

Test Day

Eat a healthy breakfast the morning of your test to boost your energy levels. Taking deep breaths and focusing on positive thoughts can also help to calm your nerves. Arrive early for the exam and be prepared with any questions or materials you may need. During the exam, stay focused and take your time. Don't rush your answers and don't be afraid to ask for help if you are struggling. Take breaks to cool off your mind and return to your exam. Finally, pat yourself on the back for a job well done and relax afterwards. Celebrate your successes and recognize the hard work you have put in. Take some time to do an activity that you enjoy and reflect on what you have achieved. Finally, don't forget to take the time to rest and recharge. Feel free to call me with news of your success.
SUCESS IS YOURS WITH GOD ALMIGHTY!

Review Course Tracker/study notes

Assignment	Chapters	Topics Covered	Questions	Grades

Review Course Tracker/study notes

Assignment	Chapters	Topics Covered	Questions	Grades

REVIEW NOTES

REVIEW NOTES

REVIEW NOTES

JACKS NCLEX REVIEW

REVIEW NOTES

REVIEW NOTES

REVIEW NOTES

REVIEW NOTES

REVIEW NOTES

REVIEW NOTES

REVIEW NOTES

REVIEW NOTES

REVIEW NOTES

JACKS NCLEX REVIEW

REVIEW NOTES

REVIEW NOTES

REVIEW NOTES

REVIEW NOTES

REVIEW NOTES

REVIEW NOTES

REVIEW NOTES

REVIEW NOTES

REVIEW NOTES

REVIEW NOTES

REVIEW NOTES

www.ingramcontent.com/pod-product-compliance
Lightning Source LLC
LaVergne TN
LVHW070951210926
848482LV00002B/180